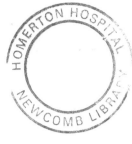

# WHO LABORATORY MANUAL

## for the examination of human semen and sperm–cervical mucus interaction

FOURTH EDITION

Published on behalf of the
WORLD HEALTH ORGANIZATION
by

1999

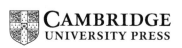

PUBLISHED BY THE PRESS SYNDICATE OF THE UNIVERSITY OF CAMBRIDGE
The Pitt Building, Trumpington Street, Cambridge, United Kingdom

CAMBRIDGE UNIVERSITY PRESS
The Edinburgh Building, Cambridge CB2 2RU, UK    http://www.cup.cam.ac.uk
40 West 20th Street, New York, NY 10011-4211, USA    http://www.cup.org
10 Stamford Road, Oakleigh, Melbourne 3166, Australia
Ruiz de Alarcón 13, 28014 Madrid, Spain

First published by Press Concern, Singapore 1980
Second edition published by Cambridge University Press 1987
Reprinted 1988, 1990
Third edition published by Cambridge University Press 1992
Reprinted 1993, 1995, 1998
Fourth edition published by Cambridge University Press 1999
Reprinted 2000

Typeset in 10.5/13pt Monotype Photina in QuarkXPress™    [SE]

*A catalogue record for this book is available from the British Library*

*Library of Congress Cataloguing in Publication data*

WHO laboratory manual for the examination of human semen and sperm
– cervical mucus interaction. – 4th ed.
    p.   cm.
Includes bibliographical references.
ISBN 0 521 64599 9 (pbk.)
1. Semen – Examination – Laboratory manuals.    2. Cervix mucus –
Examination – Laboratory manuals.    3. Sperm–ovum interactions –
Laboratory manuals.    I. World Health Organization.    II. Title:
Laboratory manual for the examination of human semen and sperm
– cervical mucus interaction.
[DNLM:    1. Semen – chemistry laboratory manuals.    2. Spermatozoa –
chemistry laboratory manuals.    3. Cervix mucus – chemistry
laboratory manuals.    4. Sperm–Ovum Interactions laboratory manuals.
QY 190 W628 1999]
RB54.W48    1999
612.6′1–dc21    98-46890 CIP
DNLM/DLC
for Library of Congress

ISBN 0 521 64599 9 paperback

Prepared by the WHO Special Programme of Research, Development and
Research Training in Human Reproduction.

# Contents

# Acknowledgements

The UNDP/UNFPA/WHO/World Bank Special Programme of Research, Development and Research Training in Human Reproduction wishes to acknowledge the participation, in the preparation and editing of the fourth edition of the *WHO Laboratory Manual for the Examination of Human Semen and Sperm–Cervical Mucus Interaction*, of the following:

**Dr R. J. Aitken**
MRC Reproductive Biology Unit
Centre for Reproductive Biology
37 Chalmers Street
Edinburgh EH3 9EW
United Kingdom

**Dr H. W. G. Baker**
University of Melbourne
Royal Women's Hospital
Department of Obstetrics and
Gynaecology
Carlton 3053, Victoria
Australia

**Dr C. L. R. Barratt**
University Department of Obstetrics
and Gynaecology
Birmingham Women's Hospital
Edgbaston
Birmingham B15 2TG
United Kingdom

**Dr H. M. Behre**
Institute of Reproductive Medicine of
the University
Domagkstrasse 11
D-48129 Münster
Germany

**Dr F. Comhaire**
Dienst Voor Inwendige Ziekten
Endocrinologie-Stofwisselingsziekten
De Pintelaan 185
9000 Gent
Belgium

**Dr T. G. Cooper**
Institute of Reproductive Medicine of
the University
Domagkstrasse 11
D-48129 Münster
Germany

**Dr C. De Jonge**
Department of Obstetrics &
Gynaecology
University of Nebraska Medical
Center
600 South 42 Street,
Omaha, NE 68198-3255
United States of America

**Dr R. Eliasson**
Head, Andrology Unit
Sophiahemmet Hospital
SE 114 86 Stockholm
Sweden

**Dr T. M. M. Farley**
UNDP/UNFPA/WHO/World Bank
Special Programme of Research,
Development and Research Training
in Human Reproduction
World Health Organization
1211 Geneva 27
Switzerland

**Mr P. D. Griffin**
UNDP/UNFPA/WHO/World Bank
Special Programme of Research,
Development and Research Training
in Human Reproduction
World Health Organization
1211 Geneva 27
Switzerland

**Dr I. Huhtaniemi**
Department of Physiology
University of Turku
Kiinamyllynkatu 10
SF-20520 Turku
Finland

**Dr T. F. Kruger**
Reproductive Biology Unit
Tygerberg Hospital
PO Box 19058
Tygerberg 7505
South Africa

**Dr M. T. Mbizvo**
Department of Obstetrics and
Gynaecology
University of Zimbabwe
PO Box A 178
Avondale
Harare
Zimbabwe

**Dr J. W. Overstreet**
Division of Reproductive Biology
Department of Obstetrics &
Gynaecology
One Shields Avenue
University of California, Davis
Davis, CA 95616
United States of America

**Mrs L. Sellaro,**
UNDP/UNFPA/WHO/World Bank
Special Programme of Research,
Development and Research Training
in Human Reproduction
World Health Organization
1211 Geneva 27
Switzerland

**Dr J. Suominen**
Department of Anatomy
University of Turku
Kiinamyllynkatu 10
SF-20520 Turku
Finland

**Dr G. M. H. Waites**
c/o Clinique de Stérilité et
d'Endocrinologie Gynécologique
Hôpital Cantonal
Universitaire de Genève
20 rue Alcide Jentzer
1211 Geneva 14
Switzerland

**Dr C. C. L. Wang**
Clinical Study Center (Box 16)
Harbor-UCLA Medical Center
1000 West Carson Street
Torrance, CA 90509
United States of America

# Abbreviations

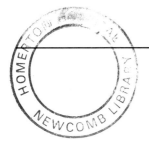

| | |
|---|---|
| BSA | bovine serum albumin (Cohn fraction V) |
| CASA | computer-aided sperm analysis |
| DMSO | dimethyl sulfoxide |
| DTT | dithiothreitol |
| EDTA | ethylenediaminetetraacetic acid |
| EQA | external quality assessment |
| HIV | human immunodeficiency virus |
| HOPT | hamster oocyte penetration test |
| HOS | hypo-osmotic swelling test |
| HPF | high-power field |
| HSA | human serum albumin (Cohn fraction V) |
| IBT | immunobead test |
| IQC | internal quality control |
| IU | international unit |
| IVF | in vitro fertilization |
| MAR | mixed antiglobulin reaction |
| MAI | multiple anomalies index |
| PAS | periodic acid Schiff |
| PBS | phosphate buffered saline |
| PCT | post-coital test |
| QC | quality control |
| ROS | reactive oxygen species |
| SCMC | sperm–cervical mucus contact |
| SDI | sperm deformity index |
| SPA | sperm penetration assay (synonymous with HOPT) |
| TZI | teratozoospermia index |
| U | (international) unit |
| WBC | white blood cell (leukocyte) |

# 1 Introduction

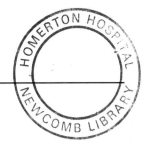

In response to a growing need for the standardization of procedures for the examination of human semen, the World Health Organization (WHO) first published a *Laboratory Manual for the Examination of Human Semen and Semen–Cervical Mucus Interaction* in 1980. The second and third editions of the manual followed in 1987 and 1992. These publications have been used extensively by clinicians and researchers worldwide. Indeed, the third edition was translated into the following languages: Arabic, Chinese, French, German, Indonesian, Italian, Portuguese and Spanish. However, the field of andrology has continued to advance rapidly, and this, together with increased awareness of the need for standardized measurements of all semen variables, has prompted the present revision.

This fourth edition comes at a time of new developments and concerns. The landmark demonstration of contraceptive efficacy with hormonally induced suppression of spermatogenesis (World Health Organization Task Force on Methods for the Regulation of Male Fertility, 1990, 1996) should lead to the development of practical, efficient and safer hormonal methods of male fertility regulation. Advances in understanding the genetic basis of male infertility, together with the successes of assisted reproductive technology, including intracytoplasmic sperm injection, have regenerated interest in the field and brought hope for men previously considered infertile. These advances in male subfertility treatment have also led to a resurgence of interest in the assessment of sperm function. Reports of declining sperm counts and increasing incidence of urogenital abnormalities and testicular cancer in some regions of the world have aroused public concern. The deterioration of semen quality is not geographically uniform as shown by studies in Denmark, Finland, France, the United Kingdom and the United States of America. Government environmental agencies and national and international scientific societies, as well as WHO, have conducted discussions on this topic without a clear consensus emerging. Further studies, perhaps on varied populations in areas with and without known environmental pollutants or toxins, are in progress. The advances in male contraceptive development and in the treatment of male subfertility, together with increasing concerns about the environment and putative consequences on male reproductive function, add fresh urgency to the search for new methods to achieve better standardization and improvement of semen analysis.

For these reasons, the UNDP/UNFPA/WHO/World Bank Special Programme of Research, Development and Research Training in Human Reproduction, after seeking advice from experts throughout the world via letters, journals and national andrology societies, formed a working group (see Acknowledgements) to revise the manual. The present edition is a companion to the *WHO Manual for the Standardized Investigation and Diagnosis of the Infertile Couple* published in 1993 by the Cambridge University Press.

Chapter 2 of the present manual, which deals with the examination of human semen, is divided into three major parts. The first part describes procedures that are considered to be essential in semen evaluation (Section 2A, 2.1 to 2.6). The second part comprises procedures considered by most laboratories to be optional but which may be of clinical diagnostic value (Section 2B, 2.7 to 2.12). The third part (Section 2C, 2.13 and 2.14) includes methods that assess sperm functional capacity and developments in computer-aided analyses for sperm morphology. These techniques may not be available in all laboratories but may be of value in the assessment of male subfertility, in reproductive toxicology studies or as research tools. In the standard procedure section describing sperm morphology, this manual recommends the Papanicolaou stain as the preferred method and the use of a simplified classification of sperm morphology according to the so-called 'strict criteria'. Computer-aided sperm analysis (CASA) for sperm motion and the zona-free hamster oocyte test have been included in the section of optional tests, as these tests may have some diagnostic applications. The section on research tests has been rewritten and updated to reflect the current consensus on the assessment of sperm functional capacity. The statistical basis of counting errors involved in semen analysis has been added and the chapter on quality control has been expanded to include discussions on practical methods of implementing quality control in any andrology laboratory.

In Appendix I, reference values of semen variables are listed. It should be noted that it is not the purpose of the manual to establish the minimum or lowest semen values compatible with achieving a pregnancy, in vivo or in vitro. It proved difficult to reach agreement on some aspects of the assessment of sperm morphology and on the provision of reference ranges since morphology assessment remains subjective. Reference ranges for human semen present some conceptual difficulties. The relationship of semen quality to fertility is complicated by many other factors, including female fertility. Thus men with abnormal semen may still be fertile while men with better than average semen quality produce pregnancies at higher than average rates. This manual is not designed only for laboratories that deal with subfertile couples. It also addresses the needs of laboratories investigating methods for male contraception and studies of reproductive toxicology. In this context, it is important for this manual to give reference values based on multicentre population studies of normal men and not the minimum requirements for fertilization. In addition, this manual suggests that it is preferable for each laboratory to determine its own reference ranges for each variable (e.g., with samples evaluated for men who have recently achieved a pregnancy).

Finally, it should be emphasized that the major purpose of this manual is to encourage the use of standard procedures to establish reference values (previously called 'normal' values) for semen analysis. This will permit improved comparability of results between laboratories and the amalgamation of data from different sources for analysis. Attention to the details of standard procedures should also sharpen the precision of results and their reproducibility. Above all, the prime objective of the earlier editions has remained: to provide a laboratory manual that will serve the needs of researchers and clinicians in developing countries.

# 2 Collection and examination of human semen

Normal semen is a mixture of spermatozoa suspended in secretions from the testis and epididymis which, at the time of ejaculation, are combined with secretions from the prostate, seminal vesicles, and bulbourethral glands. The final composition is a viscous fluid that comprises the ejaculate.

Measurements made on the whole population of ejaculated spermatozoa cannot define the fertilizing capacity of the few that reach the site of fertilization. Nevertheless, semen analysis provides essential information on the clinical status of the individual. Clearly, the collection and analysis of semen must be undertaken by properly standardized procedures if the results are to provide valid information, and this chapter and its associated Appendices (III–XVII) offer methods for this purpose. These methods are divided into standard, optional, and research procedures.

## 2A STANDARD PROCEDURES

The tests described in this part of the manual are accepted procedures that constitute the essential steps in semen evaluation.

## 2.1 Sample collection and delivery

The subject should be given clear, written or oral instructions concerning the collection and, if required, transport of the semen sample (see Appendix XIII).

(a) The sample should be collected after a minimum of 48 hours but not longer than seven days of sexual abstinence. To reduce the variability of semen analysis results, the number of days of sexual abstinence should be as constant as possible. The name of the man, the period of abstinence, the date and time of collection, completeness of collection, difficulties in producing the sample, the interval between collection and analysis should be recorded on the form accompanying each semen analysis (see Appendix XIII).

(b) Two samples should be collected for initial evaluation. The interval between the two collections should not be less than 7 days or more than 3 weeks. If the results of these two assessments are markedly different, additional samples should be examined because the results of a man's semen analysis can vary considerably (Fig. 2.1).

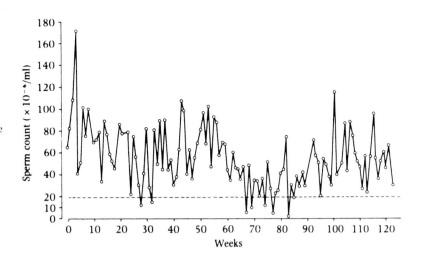

Fig. 2.1. Sperm concentrations in the semen of one man collected biweekly over 120 weeks. During this period the man received no medication and experienced no febrile illness. The dotted line indicates $20 \times 10^6$/ml (see Appendix 1A). The data illustrate the marked variations in sperm concentration that can occur in the semen of some men. (Unpublished data from C.A. Paulsen.)

(c) Ideally, the sample should be collected in a private room near the laboratory. If this is not possible, it should be delivered to the laboratory within 1 hour of collection. When the motility of the spermatozoa is abnormally low (less than 25% of spermatozoa showing rapid, progressive motility, see Section 2.4.3), the interval between collection and analysis of the second sample should be as short as possible because motility declines with time (Eliasson, 1981). If tests of sperm function are to be performed, it is critical that the spermatozoa be separated from the seminal plasma within one hour of ejaculation (see Appendix XVIII).

(d) The sample should be obtained by masturbation and ejaculated into a clean, wide-mouthed container made of glass or plastic. It should be warm (20–40 °C) to avoid reduction in sperm motility and from a batch that has been checked for toxic effects on sperm motility (see Appendix XXII). If a microbiological analysis is to be done, the subject should pass urine and then wash and rinse his hands and penis before ejaculating into a sterile container (see Section 2.9).

(e) When circumstances prevent collection by masturbation, special condoms are available for semen collection (Milex products Inc., Chicago, Illinois 60631, USA; Male Factor Pack[R], Hygiene[R], FertiPro N.V., Belgium). Ordinary latex condoms must not be used for semen collection because they interfere with the viability of the spermatozoa. *Coitus interruptus* is not acceptable as a means of collection because the first portion of the ejaculate, which usually contains the highest concentration of spermatozoa, may be lost. Moreover, there will be cellular and bacteriological contamination of the sample and the acid pH of the vaginal fluid adversely affects sperm motility.

(f) It is important to emphasize to the subject that the semen sample should be complete.

(g)   The sample should be protected from extremes of temperature (less than 20 °C and more than 40 °C) during transport to the laboratory.

(h)   The container must be adequately labelled with the subject's name (and/or identification number) and with the date and time of collection.

## 2.2   Safe handling of specimens

Laboratory technicians should be aware that semen samples may contain harmful infectious agents (e.g., viruses causing acquired immunodeficiency syndrome, hepatitis, and herpes simplex) and should therefore be handled as a biohazard with extreme care. If semen culture is to be performed or the sample is to be processed for bioassays, intrauterine insemination, or in vitro fertilization, sterile materials and techniques must be used in handling the samples. Safety guidelines as outlined in Appendix II should be strictly observed. Good laboratory practice is fundamental to laboratory safety (WHO, 1983).

## 2.3   Initial macroscopic examination

### 2.3.1   Liquefaction

A normal semen sample liquefies within 60 minutes at room temperature, although usually this occurs within 15 minutes. In some cases, complete liquefaction does not occur within 60 minutes, and this should be recorded. Normal semen samples may contain jelly-like grains (gelatinous bodies) which do not liquefy and do not appear to have any clinical significance. The presence of mucous streaks may interfere with semen analysis.

The sample must be well mixed in the original container and must not be shaken vigorously. During liquefaction, continuous gentle mixing or rotation of the sample container may reduce errors in determining sperm concentration (de Ziegler et al., 1987). If sperm motility is to be assessed at 37 °C, the sample should be equilibrated to this temperature during liquefaction and mixing.

Occasionally, samples may not liquefy, in which case additional treatment, mechanical mixing or enzyme digestion (e.g., bromelain 1 g/l) may be necessary. Some samples can also be induced to liquefy by the addition of an equal volume of medium followed by repeated pipetting. All these manipulations may affect seminal plasma biochemistry, sperm motility and sperm morphology and their use must be recorded.

### 2.3.2   Appearance

The semen sample should be examined immediately after liquefaction or within one hour of ejaculation, first by simple inspection at room temperature. A normal sample has a homogenous, grey–opalescent appearance. It may appear less opaque if the sperm concentration is very low, red–brown when red blood cells are present or yellow in a patient with jaundice or taking some vitamins.

### 2.3.3 Volume

The volume of the ejaculate may be measured using a graduated cylinder with a conical base or by weighing standard containers with and without semen. Plastic syringes should not be used because they may affect sperm motility and hypodermic needles are unsafe.

### 2.3.4 Viscosity

The viscosity (sometimes referred to as 'consistency') of the liquefied sample should be recognized as being different from coagulation. It can be estimated by gentle aspiration into a wide-bore 5-ml pipette and then allowing the semen to drop by gravity and observing the length of the thread. A normal sample leaves the pipette as small discrete drops. In cases of abnormal viscosity the drop will form a thread more than 2 cm long. Alternatively, the viscosity may be evaluated by introducing a glass rod into the sample and observing the length of the thread that forms on withdrawal of the rod. Again, the thread should not exceed 2 cm.

High viscosity can interfere with determinations of sperm motility, concentration and antibody coating of spermatozoa. The methods to reduce viscosity are the same as those for delayed liquefaction (see Section 2.3.1.).

### 2.3.5 pH

The pH should be measured at a uniform time within one hour of ejaculation. A drop of semen is spread evenly onto the pH paper (range: pH 6.1 to 10.0 or 6.4 to 8.0). After 30 seconds, the colour of the impregnated zone should be uniform and is compared with the calibration strip to read the pH. Whatever type of pH paper is used for this analysis, its accuracy should be checked against known standards.

If the pH is less than 7.0 in a sample with azoospermia, there may be obstruction of the ejaculatory ducts or bilateral congenital absence of the vasa.

## 2.4 Initial microscopic investigation

During the initial microscopic investigation of the sample, estimates are made of the concentration, motility, agglutination of spermatozoa, and presence of cellular elements other than spermatozoa.

A phase-contrast microscope is recommended for all examinations of unstained preparations of fresh semen or washed spermatozoa. An ordinary light microscope can be used for unstained preparations, particularly if the condenser is lowered to disperse the light.

### 2.4.1 Preparation for routine semen analysis

The volume of semen and the dimensions of the coverslip must be standardized so that the analyses are always carried out in a preparation of fixed depth of about 20 μm. This allows a rough estimate of sperm concentration to be made in order to determine how to prepare the semen for the accurate determination of sperm concentration. Depths less than 20 μm may constrain the rotational movement of spermatozoa.

A fixed volume of 10 μl semen is delivered onto a clean glass slide with a positive displacement pipette and covered with a 22 mm × 22 mm coverslip. The weight of the coverslip spreads the sample for optimum viewing and care should be taken to avoid forming and trapping bubbles between the coverslip and the slide.

The freshly made wet preparation is left to stabilize for approximately one minute. Since sperm motility and velocity are highly dependent on temperature, the assessment of motility should preferably be performed at 37 °C, using a warmed stage. The examination may be carried out at room temperature, between 20 and 24 °C, but temperature must be standardized in the laboratory as it will affect the classification of the grades of motility. Initial evaluation at 100× total magnification (i.e., 10× objective and 10× ocular) provides an overview for determining mucus strand formation, sperm aggregation, and the evenness of spread of spermatozoa on the slide. The preparation is then examined at a magnification of 400× total magnification.

### 2.4.2 Preliminary estimation of sperm concentration

With different microscopes the 400× magnification field of view varies in diameter, usually in the range between 250 and 400 μm corresponding to 1 to 2.5 nl with a 20 μm depth of sample. The diameter of the field can be determined with a micrometer or the grid of a counting chamber. Scanning the slide and estimating the number of spermatozoa per field or part of a field equivalent to 1 nl gives an approximate sperm concentration in $10^6$/ml. This estimate is used to decide the dilution for determining the sperm concentration by haemocytometry: <15 spermatozoa, dilution 1:5; 15–40 spermatozoa, dilution 1:10; 40–200 spermatozoa, dilution 1:20; >200 spermatozoa, dilution 1:50 (see Table 2.1).

If the number of spermatozoa per visual field varies considerably, it indicates that the sample is not homogeneous. In such cases, the semen sample should be mixed again thoroughly. Lack of homogeneity may also result from abnormal consistency, abnormal liquefaction,

Table 2.1. *Dilutions and conversion factors for the improved Neubauer haemocytometer*

| Spermatozoa per 400×field | Dilution (semen+diluent) | Conversion factors Number of large squares counted | | |
| --- | --- | --- | --- | --- |
| | | 25 | 10 | 5 |
| <15 | 1:5 (1+4) | 20 | 8 | 4 |
| 15–40 | 1:10 (1+9) | 10 | 4 | 2 |
| 40–200 | 1:20 (1+19) | 5 | 2 | 1 |
| >200 | 1:50 (1+49) | 2 | 0.8 | 0.4 |

aggregation of spermatozoa in mucous threads, or from sperm agglutination. These abnormalities should be mentioned in the semen analysis report.

If the number of spermatozoa is low (<1–2/field, 400× magnification), it is possible to determine the sperm concentration after centrifugation to concentrate the sample. One millilitre of semen (or as much of the ejaculate as possible) is centrifuged at 600$g$ for 15 minutes. A known volume of the seminal plasma is then removed and the remainder is thoroughly mixed and counted as described in Section 2.5.2. The final concentration is corrected to include the volume of the supernatant removed. Sperm motility and morphology assessments can also be performed on the sample after centrifugation. If the number of spermatozoa is low (<1–2/field), it is sufficient for clinical purposes to report the concentration as <2 × 10$^6$/ml with a note on whether or not motile spermatozoa were seen.

All samples in which no spermatozoa are detected by microscopy should be centrifuged to detect the presence of spermatozoa in the sediment. Centrifugation at >3000$g$ for 15 minutes is recommended. Only when no spermatozoa are found after a complete and systematic search of all of the resuspended precipitate should samples be classified as azoospermic.

### 2.4.3 Assessment of sperm motility

A simple grading system is recommended which provides an assessment of sperm motility without the need for complex equipment. Other methods of assessment of sperm motility, including computer-aided sperm analysis (CASA), are given in Section 2.11.

At least five microscopic fields are assessed in a systematic way to classify 200 spermatozoa (Fig. 2.2). The motility of each spermatozoon is graded 'a', 'b', 'c', or 'd', according to whether it shows:

a. rapid progressive motility (i.e., ≥25μm/s at 37°C and ≥20 μm/s at 20°C; note that 25 μm is approximately equal to five head lengths or half a tail length);

Fig. 2.2. (*a*) Tramlines in the field of view of the microscope to aid assessment of sperm motility. (*b*) Systematic selection of eight fields for assessment of sperm motility at least 5 mm from the edges of the cover slip.

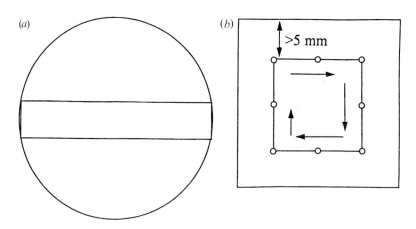

(*a*)

(*b*)

>5 mm

b.    slow or sluggish progressive motility;

c.    nonprogressive motility ($<5$ μm/s);

d.    immotility.

Within a defined area of the field indicated by lines (Fig. 2.2(*a*) and (*b*)) formed by a graticule in the focal plane of the microscope, or in the whole field if the sperm concentration is low, all spermatozoa with grade a and b motility are counted first. Subsequently spermatozoa with nonprogressive motility (grade c) and immotile spermatozoa (grade d) are counted in the same area. The number of spermatozoa in each category can be tallied with the aid of a laboratory counter. The count of 200 spermatozoa is repeated on a separate 10μl specimen from the same semen sample and the percentages in each motility grade from the two independent counts are compared. Figure 2.3 shows the range of differences between the percentages that are expected to occur in 95% of samples due to counting error alone. Larger differences would suggest that miscounting had occurred or that the spermatozoa were not randomly distributed on the slide. In this case two new slides should be prepared and sperm motility reassessed.

### 2.4.4    *Cellular elements other than spermatozoa*

The ejaculate invariably contains cells other than spermatozoa collectively referred to as 'round cells'. These include epithelial cells from the genitourinary tract, prostate cells, spermatogenic cells, and leukocytes (see Fig. 2.4). As a general guide, a normal ejaculate should not contain more than $5 \times 10^6$ round cells/ml.

*Leukocytes* Leukocytes, predominantly neutrophils, are present in most human ejaculates (Tomlinson et al., 1993). Excessive numbers of these cells (*leukocytospermia*) may be associated with infection and

Fig. 2.3. Approximate 95% confidence interval ranges for differences between two percentages determined from duplicate counts of 100, 200 or 400 spermatozoa. To assess the percentages from two counts of 200, calculate their average and difference. If the difference is greater than indicated by the N=200 curve, the sample must be reanalysed. The lower curve shows the increase in precision for two assessments of 400 spermatozoa (N=400). For an average result of 5%, the 95% confidence interval is 3%. The large statistical counting errors associated with counting only 100 spermatozoa are apparent from the top curve (N=100). For a result of 5%, the two single assessments of 100 spermatozoa could be 3% and 9% by chance alone. (See Appendix XXII for a larger version of this graph.)

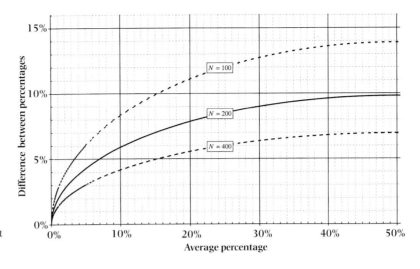

*Example 1:*
Sperm motility in duplicate counts of 200 spermatozoa are: grade a = 3% and 20%; b = 32% and 40%; c = 5% and 5%; and d = 60% and 35%. The most common category is grade d motility (60% and 35%), with average 47.5% and difference 25%. From Fig. 2.3 it can be seen that, for N = 200 spermatozoa in each sample, and for an average of 47.5%, a difference of up to 10% would be expected to occur by chance but a difference of 25% would not. Thus the results are discarded and a fresh preparation estimated. Note that, if the percentage difference of one grade of motility is larger than expected, then often that of another grade is also larger, as here for grade a. Only the difference in the percentages of the most common grade need be compared.

*Example 2:*
Sperm motility in duplicate counts of 200 spermatozoa are: grade a = 32% and 25%; b = 4% and 3%; c = 4% and 4% and d = 60% and 68%. The most common category is grade d, with average 64% and difference 8%. Since the average percentage 64% is not in Fig. 2.3, the expected difference for an average percentage 36% (= 100%–64%) is looked up. For N = 200 in each sample, differences up to 9.5% occur by chance alone and the observed difference is less than this. The mean percentages for each grade are calculated: 28.5%, 3.5%, 4%, and 64%. Note that the convention is to round 0.5% to the nearest *even* number, i.e., 28.5% *down* to 28% but 3.5% *up* to 4%. The percentages reported should add up to 100% by adjusting the most common group if necessary, i.e., a = 28%, b = 4%, c = 4% and d = 64%.

poor sperm quality (Wolff et al., 1990). The number of leukocytes should not exceed $1 \times 10^6$/ ml.

Several techniques have been devised for quantifying the leukocyte population in semen. Two cytochemical techniques based on the presence of intracellular peroxidase and on leukocyte-specific antigens are given in Appendix III. The peroxidase technique (Fig. 2.4*a*) gives

Fig. 2.4. Leukocytes in human semen (400×). (*a*) Stained with the peroxidase method. (From C. De Jonge; see Appendix III.1.) (*b*) Stained with a monoclonal antibody against the common leukocyte antigen CD45 (see Appendix III.2).

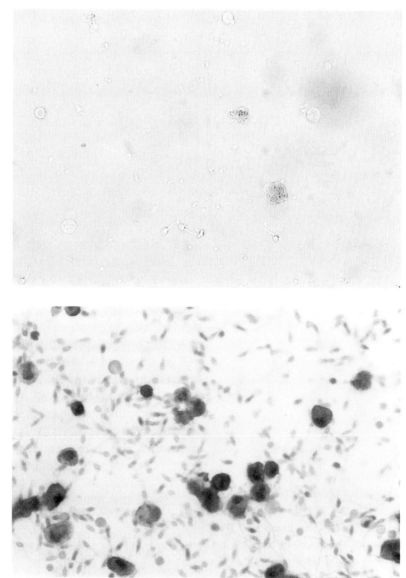

(*a*)

(*b*)

estimates that are lower than those obtained using pan-leukocyte monoclonal antibodies (Fig. 2.4*b*).

When the number of leukocytes in semen is high, microbiological tests should be performed to investigate if there is an accessory gland infection. Such tests include the examination of the first voided urine, the second voided urine, the expressed prostatic fluid, and the post-prostatic massage urine (Meares & Stamey, 1972). They also include the biochemical analysis of seminal plasma, since infection of the accessory glands often causes abnormal secretory function (Section 2.10; Comhaire et al., 1980). However the absence of leukocytes does not exclude the possibility of an accessory gland infection (see World Health Organization, 1993).

*Immature germ cells* The round cells other than leukocytes include round spermatids, spermatocytes, spermatogonia, and exfoliated epithelial cells. These are often degenerating and difficult to identify.

The different types of immature germ cells appearing in semen (Fig. 2.11) are usually indicative of disorders of spermatogenesis; their identification can be aided by the use of the Bryan–Leishman stain (see Appendix VIII of the third edition of this manual). They may be distinguished from leukocytes by their cytological features and the absence of intracellular peroxidase and lack of leukocyte-specific antigens (see Appendix III). Round spermatids may be identified by staining the developing acrosome, e.g., with periodic acid Schiff stain. Excessive shedding of immature germ cells usually results from impaired seminiferous tubule function as in hypospermatogenesis, varicocele, and Sertoli cell dysfunction and is associated with reduced success of in vitro fertilization (Tomlinson et al., 1992).

*Counting cells other than spermatozoa* The concentration of such cells can be estimated in wet preparations using a suitable haemocytometer in the same way as spermatozoa (see Section 2.5.2). Since only spermatozoa are included in the sperm count, the concentration of other types of germ cells or leukocytes can be calculated relative to that of spermatozoa. If $N$ is the number of a given cell type counted in the same field(s) as 100 spermatozoa and $S$ is the sperm concentration in millions/ml, then the concentration $C$ of the given cell type in millions/ml can be calculated from the formula

$$C = \frac{N \times S}{100}$$

For example, if the number of immature germ cells or leukocytes counted is 10 per 100 spermatozoa and the sperm count is $120 \times 10^6$/ml, the concentration of such cells is

$$\frac{10 \times 120 \times 10^6}{100} \text{ per millilitre} = 12 \text{ million per ml.}$$

If no cells are seen for the whole slide, it is appropriate to report that there are fewer than 3.7 cells/unit volume examined (the upper 95% confidence limits of 0 is 3.7 in the Poisson distribution). Thus for a $1\,\mu l$ sample the count is $<3700$ cells/ml, which is the lower limit of detection. The counting errors are large when only a few leukocytes are seen. In research studies of seminal leukocytes or other cells, larger volumes of semen are needed to count 200 cells of interest in order to achieve acceptably low counting errors (see Section 2.5.2).

### 2.4.5 Agglutination

Agglutination of spermatozoa means that motile spermatozoa stick to each other head to head, tail to tail or in a mixed way, e.g., head to tail. The adherence either of immotile spermatozoa to each other or of motile spermatozoa to mucous threads, cells other than spermatozoa, or debris is considered to be nonspecific aggregation rather than agglutination and should be recorded as such.

The presence of agglutination is suggestive of, but not sufficient evidence for, an immunological cause of infertility. Agglutination is assessed at the time of determining sperm motility. The type of agglutination should be recorded, e.g., head to head, tail to tail or mixed. A semiquantitative grading from − (no agglutination) to +++ (severe clumping in which all the motile spermatozoa are agglutinated), can be used.

## 2.5 Further microscopic examinations

### 2.5.1 Sperm vitality by dye exclusion

Sperm vitality is reflected in the proportion of spermatozoa that are 'alive' as determined by either dye exclusion or hypo-osmotic swelling (see Section 2.8). This should be determined if the percentage of immotile spermatozoa exceeds 50%. The proportion of live spermatozoa can be determined by using staining techniques that are based on the principle that dead cells with a damaged plasma membrane take up certain stains. Details of the protocols for performing these techniques are given in Appendix IV.

Two hundred spermatozoa are counted with the light or phase-contrast microscope, differentiating the live (unstained) spermatozoa from the dead (stained) cells.

Sperm vitality assessments provide a check on the accuracy of the motility evaluation, since the percentage of dead cells should not exceed (within counting error) the percentage of immotile spermatozoa. The presence of a large proportion of vital but immotile cells may be indicative of structural defects in the flagellum.

### 2.5.2 Assessment of sperm concentration

The concentration of spermatozoa should be determined using the haemocytometer method on two separate preparations of the semen sample, one for each side of the counting chamber. The dilution is determined (1:5, 1:10, 1:20, 1:50) from the preliminary estimation of sperm concentration (Section 2.4.2). For example, a 1:20 dilution is made by diluting 5 µl of liquefied semen with 95 µl of diluent. The diluent is prepared by adding to distilled water 50 g sodium bicarbonate ($NaHCO_3$), 10 ml 35% (v/v) formalin, and either 0.25 g trypan blue (Colour Index C.I. 23850) or 5 ml saturated aqueous

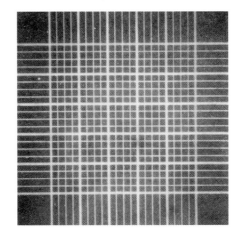

Fig. 2.5. The central grid of the improved Neubauer haemocytometer contains 25 squares in which the spermatozoa are to be counted (see Section 2.5.2 and Table 2.1).

gentian violet, and making up the solution to a final volume of 1 litre. The stain need not be included if phase-contrast microscopy is used.

White-blood-cell pipettes and automatic pipettes relying upon air displacement are not accurate enough for making volumetric dilutions of semen. A positive-displacement type of pipette should be used (see Appendix XXII).

Secure the coverslip on the counting chambers of the improved Neubauer haemocytometer by lightly wetting either side of the wells (use a drop of water on the finger). Press the coverslip firmly onto the chambers so that iridescence (Newton's rings) is observed between the two glass surfaces. Transfer approximately 10 µl of the thoroughly mixed diluted specimen from each duplicate dilution to each of the counting chambers of the haemocytometer. This is done by carefully touching the edge of the cover glass with the pipette tip and allowing each chamber to fill by capillary action. The chambers should not be over or underfilled and the cover glass should not be moved. The haemocytometer is allowed to stand for about five minutes in a humid chamber to prevent drying out. The cells sediment during this time and are then counted, preferably with a phase-contrast microscope, at a magnification of 200 to 400×. The count should be made of complete spermatozoa (heads with tails). Defective spermatozoa (pinheads and tailless heads) should also be counted but recorded separately.

The procedure for counting the spermatozoa in the haemocytometer chamber is as follows. The central square of the grid in an improved Neubauer haemocytometer contains 25 large squares, each containing 16 smaller squares (Fig. 2.5). For samples containing fewer than ten spermatozoa per large square, spermatozoa in the whole grid of 25 large squares should be assessed; for samples

Fig. 2.6. Approximate 95% confidence interval for differences between two counts. To assess these counts, calculate their sum and difference. If the difference is greater than indicated by the curve there may be a systematic error (see Chapter 4) and the sample must be reanalysed. The large statistical counting errors associated with counting fewer than 200 spermatozoa are apparent. For example, for a mean count of 60 spermatozoa (sum 120), the two counts could be 50 and 70 by chance alone. (See Appendix XXII for a larger version of this graph.)

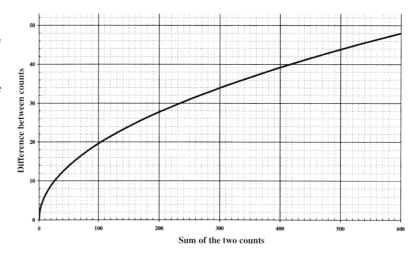

Difference between counts — Sum of the two counts

containing ten to 40 spermatozoa per large square, ten large squares should be assessed; and, for samples containing more than 40 spermatozoa per large square, spermatozoa in five large squares should be assessed. If a spermatozoon lies on the line dividing two adjacent squares, it should be counted only if it is on the upper or the left side of the square being assessed.

Duplicate counts of 200 spermatozoa must be performed to achieve an acceptably low counting error. To check the two counts, calculate their sum and difference. Figure 2.6 shows the range of differences that are expected to occur in 95% of samples from statistical counting error alone. Larger differences suggest an error of dilution, a miscounting, or a nonrandom distribution of spermatozoa in the diluted semen. When differences in counts are greater than those indicated by the curve in Fig. 2.6, two fresh duplicate dilutions of semen must be prepared and recounted.

---

*Example 1*:
The counts of ten squares in each chamber give 250 and 198 spermatozoa. The sum is 448 and the difference 52 is greater than the number expected by chance (Fig. 2.6). The results are thus discarded, the sample thoroughly remixed, dilution performed in duplicate again and each counted.

*Example 2*:
Counts of ten squares in each chamber yield 247 and 213 spermatozoa. The sum is 460 and the difference is 34. Fig. 2.6 shows that, for two counts with a total of 460 spermatozoa, differences less than 42 frequently occur by chance alone, and the observed difference is below this limit. The average count is calculated ($460/2 = 230$) and the concentration estimated from the conversion factors in Table 2.1.

---

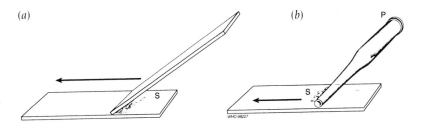

Fig. 2.7. Making smears for staining for sperm morphology. (*a*) 'Feathering' method for undiluted semen. The semen drop (S) spreads along the back edge of the angled slide and is pulled forward over the flat slide to form the smear. (*b*) Pipette method for washed samples. A drop of the suspension (S) is spread over the surface of the slide by the horizontally held pipette (P).

(*a*)

(*b*)

In order to determine the concentration of spermatozoa in the original semen sample in millions/ml, the average number of spermatozoa is divided by the appropriate conversion factor shown in Table 2.1. For example, for an average count of 230 on a 1 : 20 dilution and ten squares counted per chamber, the conversion factor is 2 and the sperm concentration $115 \times 10^6$/ml.

Chambers, other than the haemocytometer, are available for determining sperm concentration, e.g., the Makler chamber (Makler, 1980) and the Microcell (Ginsburg & Armant, 1990). Such chambers, while convenient in that they can be used without dilution of the specimen, may lack the accuracy and precision of the haemocytometer technique. When used, it is recommended that their validity be established by comparison with the haemocytometer method.

### 2.5.3 Assessment of sperm morphology

Although the morphological variability of the human spermatozoon makes sperm morphology assessment difficult, observations on spermatozoa recovered from the female reproductive tract (especially in postcoital cervical mucus) or from the surface of the zona pellucida have helped to define the appearance of a normal spermatozoon (Fredricsson & Bjork, 1977; Mortimer et al., 1982; Menkveld et al., 1990; Liu & Baker, 1992).

*Preparation of smears* At least two smears should be made from the fresh semen sample for duplicate assessment and in case of problems with staining. The slides should first be thoroughly cleaned, washed in 70% ethanol and dried, before a small drop of semen (5 to 20 μl) is applied to the slide. If the sperm concentration is over $20 \times 10^6$/ml, then 5 μl of semen can be used; if the sperm concentration is less than $20 \times 10^6$/ml, then 10 to 20 μl of semen should be used.

The 'feathering' technique (whereby the edge of a second slide is used to drag a drop of semen along the surface of the cleaned slide (Fig. 2.7(*a*)) may be used to make smears of spermatozoa, but care must be taken not to make the smears too thick. Feathering works well when viscosity is low but is often unsuitable for viscous semen. Alternatively, a drop of semen can be placed in the middle of a slide and then a second slide, face down, placed on top so that the semen spreads between them; the two slides are then gently pulled apart to make two smears simultaneously.

Sometimes good smears are difficult to prepare because of the varying viscosity of seminal plasma resulting in uneven thickness of the smear. Debris and a large amount of particulate material may cause spermatozoa to lie with their heads on edge. Thus, for low sperm concentrations or viscous or debris-laden samples, or when computer-assisted morphology is to be done, seminal plasma may be diluted and removed after centrifugation (Liu & Baker, 1992; Menkveld & Kruger, 1996). The sperm pellet is resuspended in an appropriate volume to obtain the highest sperm concentration possible, but not exceeding $80 \times 10^6$/ml. An aliquot of 0.2 to 0.5 ml of semen, depending on sperm concentration, is diluted to 10 ml with normal saline at room temperature. The tube is centrifuged at $800g$ for 10 minutes and most of the supernatant tipped off. The pellet is resuspended in the remaining saline, typically 20–40 μl, by gently tapping the tube. Then 5–10 μl of this suspension is placed on a glass microscope slide and the drop is spread across the slide with a pipette as illustrated in Fig. 2.7(b). The slide is then scanned at $400 \times$ total magnification to ensure that a smear has an even spread of spermatozoa and that there are at least 40 spermatozoa per $400 \times$ field without sperm clumping or overlapping. If the smear is too dense, a smaller volume is used or the sample is further diluted and another smear made. If the spermatozoa are too sparse on the slide, more semen is used to obtain a greater number of spermatozoa. These slides are allowed to dry in air and then fixed. The fixation procedure depends on the staining method.

*Staining methods* Papanicolaou stain is the method most widely used in andrology laboratories and is the method recommended by this manual. It gives good staining of the spermatozoa and other cells. It permits staining of the acrosomal and post-acrosomal regions of the head, the cytoplasmic droplet, the midpiece, and the tail (Appendix V and Fig. 2.9). The Shorr stain (Appendix VI and Fig. 2.10) gives similar results to those of the Papanicolaou stain for normal forms (Meschede et al., 1993). In some laboratories, a rapid staining method such as the Diff-Quik is used (Kruger et al., 1987, and Appendix VII). Some smears stained by rapid procedures may have background staining and may not always give the same quality as the Papanicolaou stain. Also, the size of the head of the spermatozoa stained by Diff-Quik is larger than that stained by Papanicolaou or Shorr stains (Kruger et al., 1988).

With these stains, the head is stained pale blue in the acrosomal region and dark blue in the post-acrosomal region. The midpiece may show some red staining. The tail is also stained blue or reddish.

Cytoplasmic droplets, usually located behind the head and around the midpiece, are stained green with the Papanicolaou stain (Fig. 2.9).

### 2.5.4 Classification of sperm morphology

The heads of stained human spermatozoa are slightly smaller than the heads of living spermatozoa in the original semen, although their shapes are not appreciably different (Katz et al., 1986). Strict criteria should be applied when assessing the morphological normality of the spermatozoon (Menkveld et al., 1990). For a spermatozoon to be considered normal, the sperm head, neck, midpiece, and tail must be normal. The head should be oval in shape. Allowing for the slight shrinkage that fixation and staining induce, the length of the head should be 4.0–5.0 μm and the width 2.5-3.5 μm. The length-to-width ratio should be 1.50 to 1.75. These ranges are the 95% confidence limits for Papanicolaou-stained sperm heads (Katz et al., 1986). Estimation of the length and width of the spermatozoon can be made with an ocular micrometer. There should be a well-defined acrosomal region comprising 40–70% of the head area. The midpiece should be slender, less than 1 μm in width, about one and a half times the length of the head, and attached axially to the head. Cytoplasmic droplets should be less than half the size of the normal head. The tail should be straight, uniform, thinner than the midpiece, uncoiled and approximately 45 μm long. This classification scheme requires that all 'borderline' forms be considered abnormal (Kruger et al., 1986; Menkveld et al., 1990). Using these criteria of classification, there are data to show the predictive value of sperm morphology for fertilization in vitro (Kruger et al., 1986, 1988; Kobayashi et al., 1991; Enginsu et al., 1991; Liu & Baker, 1992; Ombelet et al., 1995).

Since the recommended morphological assessment considers the functional regions of the spermatozoon, it is considered unnecessary routinely to distinguish between all the variations in head size and shape or between the various midpiece and tail defects. However, an additional comment should be made regarding the prevalent defects.

The following categories of defects should be noted (see examples in Figs. 2.8–2.10).

(a) *Head defects*, namely large, small, tapered, pyriform, round, and amorphous heads, vacuolated heads (>20% of the head area occupied by unstained vacuolar areas), heads with small acrosomal area (<40% of head area) and double heads, or any combination of these.

(b) *Neck and midpiece defects*, namely 'bent' neck (the neck and tail form an angle of greater than 90% to the long axis of the head), asymmetrical insertion of the midpiece into the head, thick or irregular midpiece, abnormally thin midpiece (i.e., no mitochondrial sheath), or any combination of these.

(c) *Tail defects*, namely short, multiple, hairpin, broken tails, bent tails (>90°), tails of irregular width, coiled tails, or any combination of these.

Fig. 2.8. Schematic drawings of some abnormal forms of human spermatozoa. (Adapted from Kruger et al., 1993.) (A) Head defects. (a) Tapered, (b) Pyriform, (c) Round, small and acrosome either absent, or present, (d) Amorphous, (e) Vacuolated, (f) Acrosomal area small. (B) Neck and midpiece defects. (g) Bent neck, (h) Asymmetrical insertion of midpiece, (i) Thick midpiece, (j) Thin mid-piece. (C) Tail defects. (k) Short tail, (l) Bent tail, (m) Coiled tail. (D) Cytoplasmic droplet defect. (n) Droplet greater than one third the area of the normal sperm head.

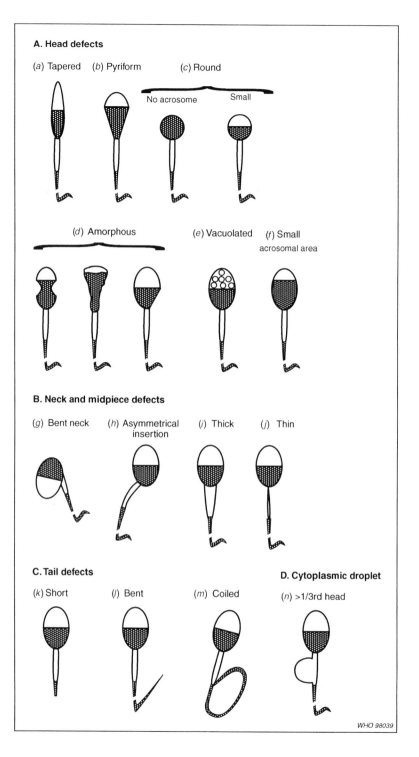

**A. Head defects**

(a) Tapered    (b) Pyriform      (c) Round

No acrosome    Small

(d) Amorphous      (e) Vacuolated    (f) Small acrosomal area

**B. Neck and midpiece defects**

(g) Bent neck    (h) Asymmetrical insertion    (i) Thick    (j) Thin

**C. Tail defects**      **D. Cytoplasmic droplet**

(k) Short    (l) Bent    (m) Coiled    (n) >1/3rd head

WHO 98039

20

Fig. 2.9. Photomicrographs (~1700×) of Papanicolaou-stained spermatozoa (From J. Suominen;. see Appendix V). (A) (1) Abnormal, large head, too wide (>3.5 μm), (2) Abnormal, vacuolated and small acrosomal area, (3) Abnormal, amorphous head, (4) Normal, (5) Abnormal, small acrosomal area, (6) Abnormal, amorphous head and cytoplasmic droplet, (7) Normal, (8) Abnormal, small acrosomal area and vacuoles.

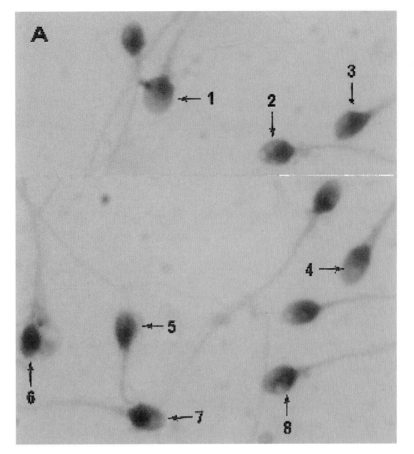

(d) *Cytoplasmic droplets* greater than one-half of the area of a normal sperm head. The droplets are usually located in the midpiece.

Only recognizable spermatozoa with a tail are considered in a differential morphology count; immature cells up to and including the round spermatid stage are not counted as spermatozoa (Fig 2.11). Loose or free sperm heads are not counted as spermatozoa but are recorded separately (see Section 2.5.2). Coiled tails may be associated with low sperm motility or indicate that the spermatozoa have been exposed to hypo-osmotic stress. Occasionally, many of the spermatozoa may have a specific structural defect such as failure of the acrosome to develop, causing the 'small round-head defect' or 'globozoospermia' (Fig 2.8). Failure of the basal plate to attach to the nucleus at the opposite pole to the acrosome causes the heads and tails to detach on spermiation. The heads are absorbed and only tails are found in the semen giving the 'pinhead' defect. Pinheads (free tails) are not counted as head defects since they only rarely possess any chromatin or head structures anterior to the basal plate. If many pinheads are seen, this should also be noted separately.

Fig. 2.9. (*cont.*)
(B) (1) Abnormal, thick mid-piece, (2) Abnormal, amorphous asymmetrical head, (3) Abnormal, asymmetrical head, (4) Abnormal, amorphous round head with asymmetrical postacrosomal region, (5) Abnormal, cytoplasmic droplet, (6) Abnormal, round head, (7) Normal (despite slight asymmetry of the head), (8) Abnormal, small head with small acrosomal area.

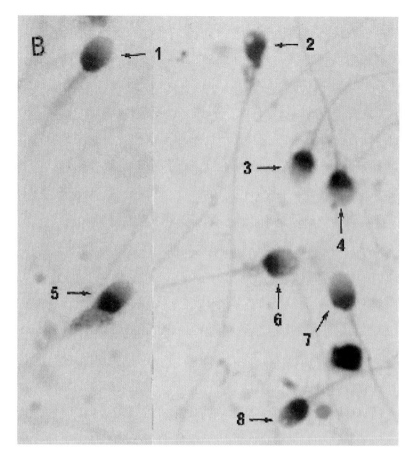

### 2.5.5 Performing a sperm morphology count

With stained preparations, a 100×oil-immersion bright-field objective and at least a 10× ocular should be used. Morphological evaluation should be performed in several systematically selected areas of the slide (Fig. 2.2(*b*)). As the slide is examined systematically from one microscopic field to another, all normal spermatozoa are assessed and scored, and the defects of the abnormal spermatozoa are noted. Overlapping spermatozoa and those lying with the head on edge cannot be assessed. The latter can be recognized by focusing up and down. It is essential to use an ocular micrometer to estimate the size of the spermatozoa. Even experienced observers should use the built-in micrometer to check sperm head size with each batch of slides to be examined.

At least 200 consecutive spermatozoa are counted (assessing 200 once is better than 100 twice). Although it is preferable to count 200 spermatozoa twice to reduce counting error and variability, it may not be practicable to do this for every sample in every laboratory. However, when the diagnosis and treatment of the patient crucially depends on

Fig. 2.9. (*cont.*)
(C) (1) Normal, (2) Abnormal, pyriform head, (3) Normal (despite slightly tapering head), (4) Abnormal, amorphous head, (5) Abnormal, small acrosomal area, thick mid-piece and asymmetrical insertion, (6) Abnormal, amorphous head with thick mid-piece.

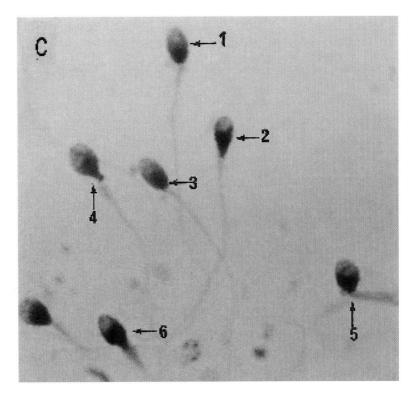

the percentage of spermatozoa with normal morphology, 200 spermatozoa should be assessed twice to increase the precision (see Fig. 2.3).

## 2.6 Testing for antibody-coating of spermatozoa

Sperm antibodies in semen belong almost exclusively to two immunoglobulin classes: IgA and IgG. IgA antibodies might have greater clinical importance than do IgG antibodies (Kremer & Jager, 1980). IgM antibodies, because of their large molecular size, are rarely found in semen.

The screening test for antibodies is performed on the fresh semen sample and makes use of either the immunobead test (IBT) (Bronson et al., 1982; Clarke et al., 1982) or the mixed antiglobulin reaction (MAR) test (for review see Bronson et al., 1984). For these tests to be valid, at least 200 motile spermatozoa must be available for counting.

The results from the immunobead test and the MAR test do not always agree (Scarselli et al., 1987; Hellstrom et al., 1989). The immunobead test correlates well with immobilization tests carried out on serum. When these tests are positive, additional tests (sperm–cervical mucus contact test, sperm–cervical mucus capillary tube test) should be done (see Chapter 5).

Fig. 2.9. (*cont.*)
(D) (1) Abnormal, small acrosomal area, too wide (length-to-width ratio <1.5) and round, (2) Abnormal, small round head, no acrosome, (3) Abnormal, small head and thick mid-piece, (4) Abnormal, round head and thick mid-piece. (E) (1) Abnormal, tapered head, (2) Abnormal, pyriform head, (3) Abnormal, nonoval amorphous head with broken neck, (4) Normal.

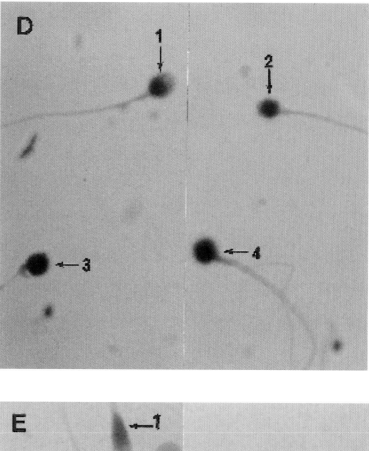

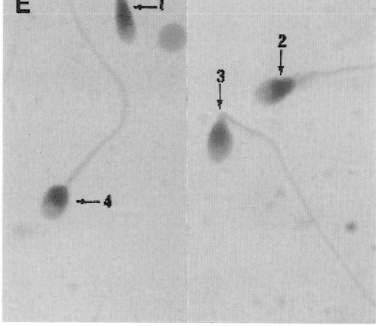

Fig. 2.9. (*cont.*)
(F) (1) Abnormal, large head and thick mid-piece, (2) Normal, (3) Normal, (4) Abnormal, vacuolated amorphous head with asymmetrical postacrosomal region, (5) Abnormal, pyriform head and vacuolated acrosomal area, (6) Abnormal, small amorphous head, (7) Abnormal, amorphous head and large cytoplasmic droplet, (8) Normal.

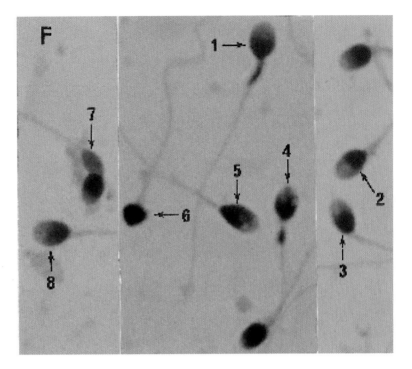

### 2.6.1 Immunobead test

Antibodies present on the sperm surface can be detected by the direct immunobead test (Appendix VIII). Immunobeads are polyacrylamide spheres with covalently bound rabbit antihuman immunoglobulins. The presence of IgG and IgA antibodies can be assessed simultaneously with this test.

Spermatozoa are washed free of seminal fluid by repeated centrifugation and resuspended in buffer. The sperm suspension is mixed with a suspension of Immunobeads. The preparation is examined at $400 \times$ magnification with a phase-contrast microscope. Immunobeads adhere to the motile spermatozoa that have surface-bound antibodies. The percentage of motile spermatozoa with surface antibodies is determined, the pattern of binding is noted and the class (IgG, IgA) of these antibodies can be identified by using different sets of Immunobeads (Appendix VIII).

Sperm penetration into the cervical mucus and in vivo fertilization tend not to be significantly impaired unless 50% or more of the motile spermatozoa have antibody bound to them (Ayvaliotis et al., 1985; Clarke et al., 1985). On this basis, at least 50% of the motile spermatozoa must be coated with Immunobeads before the test is considered to be clinically significant. Furthermore, Immunobead binding restricted to the tail tip is not associated with impaired fertility and can be present in fertile men.

Fig. 2.10.
Photomicrographs (~ 2300×) of Shorr-stained spermatozoa. (From C. Garrett & H.W.G. Baker; see Appendix VI.) (1) Abnormal, thick neck. (2) Normal. (3) Abnormal, thick neck. (4) Abnormal, amorphous, small acrosome area, thick neck. (5) Abnormal, round, small head, acrosome absent. (6) Abnormal, pyriform head, cytoplasmic droplet. (7) Abnormal, amorphous, small head, small acrosomal area, coiled tail. (8) Abnormal, pyriform head, tail absent. (9) Abnormal, amorphous. (10) Abnormal, pyriform head.

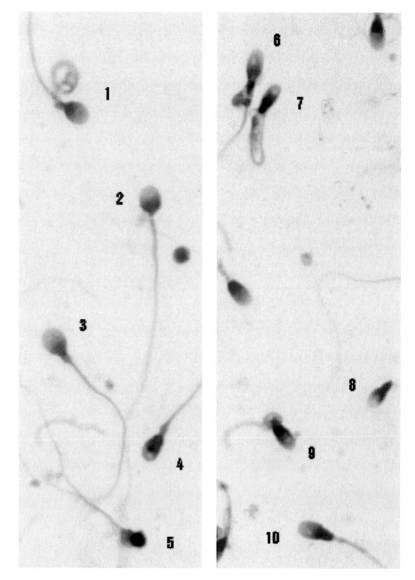

### 2.6.2 Mixed antiglobulin reaction test

The IgG and IgA MAR tests (Appendix IX) are performed by mixing fresh, untreated semen with latex particles or red blood cells coated with human IgG or IgA. To this mixture is added a monospecific anti-human-IgG antiserum. The formation of mixed agglutinates between particles and motile spermatozoa indicates the presence of IgG or IgA antibodies on the spermatozoa. The diagnosis of immunological infertility is possible when 50% or more of the motile spermatozoa have adherent particles (Barratt et al., 1992), but the diagnosis must be confirmed by sperm–mucus interaction tests (see Chapter 5).

Fig. 2.11
Photomicrographs of
Papanicolaou-stained immature
germ cells and of cells of
nontesticular origin found in
semen. (From J. Suominen.) (A)
Squamous epithelial cells ($\sim 540\times$)
(B) Two neutrophils (leukocytes)
and one monocyte ($\sim 2500\times$) (C)
Round spermatids ($\sim 1400\times$) (D)
Spermatids ($\sim 1400\times$) (E)
Macrophage ($\sim 1100\times$)

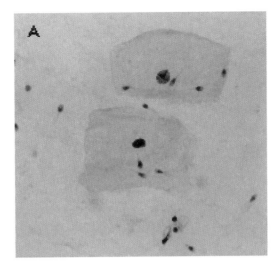

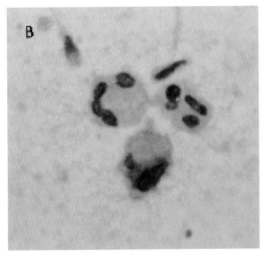

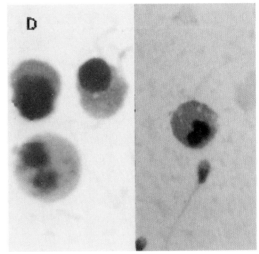

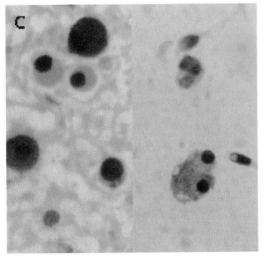

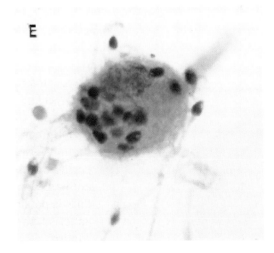

## 2B OPTIONAL TESTS

The tests in this part of the manual are not usually recommended for routine semen analysis but may be of clinical diagnostic value.

### 2.7 Calculation of indices of multiple sperm defects

Morphologically abnormal spermatozoa often have multiple defects. In earlier protocols, when multiple defects were present, only one was recorded – with priority given to defects of the sperm head over those of the midpiece and to defects of the midpiece over those of the tail. It is now customary to record the number of defects divided by the number of defective spermatozoa, a measure called the terato-zoospermia index (TZI) or multiple anomalies index (MAI) (Jouannet et al., 1988; Mortimer et al., 1990), and the number of defects divided by the total number of spermatozoa, called the sperm deformity index (SDI) (Aziz et al., 1996). These indices are predictors of sperm function both in vivo and in vitro.

A laboratory cell counter, commonly used for leukocyte counts (e.g., Clay Adams Lab Counter, Fisher Scientific, Springfield, NJ, USA, catalogue number 02-670-13) with multiple entry keys labelled 'normal', and 'head defect', 'midpiece defect', and 'tail defect', can be used. A spermatozoon with a single defect, e.g., head defect, is scored by depressing that single key and the spermatozoon is counted as one cell. A spermatozoon with head, midpiece and tail defects is scored by depressing the three appropriate keys simultaneously; the defects (total 3) in each category are counted, but the spermatozoon is counted as one cell.

Alternatively, if a cell counter is not available, a scoring sheet can be substituted. The following is an example of the calculation of indices of multiple sperm defects:

| | |
|---|---|
| Number of spermatozoa counted | 200 |
| Number of normal spermatozoa | 78 |
| Percentage of normal spermatozoa ($78/200 \times 100$) | 39% |
| Number of spermatozoa with defects ($200-78$) | 122 (61%) |
| Number with head defect | 110 (55%) |
| Number with midpiece defect | 18 (9%) |
| Number with tail defect | 16 (8%) |
| Total number of defects ($110+18+16$) | 144 |
| Teratozoospermic index (total number of defects/ number of spermatozoa with defects) $= 144/122$ | 1.18 |
| Sperm deformity index (total number of defects/ number of spermatozoa counted) $= 144/200$ | 0.72 |

The teratozoospermic index values should read between 1.00 (each abnormal spermatozoon has only one defect) to 3.00 (each abnormal spermatozoon has head, midpiece, and tail defects). Previous reports suggest that a TZI of more than 1.6 is associated with lower pregnancy rates in untreated infertile couples (Jouannet et al., 1988) and that an SDI of 1.6 is the threshold for failure of fertilization in vitro (Aziz et al., 1996).

### 2.8  Hypo-osmotic swelling (HOS) test

This is a simple test based on the semipermeability of the intact cell membrane, which causes spermatozoa to swell under hypo-osmotic conditions, when an influx of water results in an expansion of cell volume (Drevius & Eriksson, 1966). Introduced as a clinical test by Jeyendran et al. (1984), the HOS test may be used as an optional, additional vitality test. It is easy to score and gives additional information on the integrity and compliance of the cell membrane of the sperm tail. The method is given in Appendix IV.

### 2.9  Semen culture

The culture of seminal plasma to assess the presence of both aerobic and anaerobic organisms may help in the diagnosis of male accessory gland infection (Purvis & Christiansen, 1993). However, special precautions are needed to avoid contamination during the collection and handling of the semen sample for microbiological investigation. The subject should observe sexual abstinence for 5 to 7 days. Before obtaining the sample, the subject should pass urine. Immediately afterwards, he should wash his hands and penis with soap. He should rinse away the soap and dry with a fresh, clean towel. The semen container must be sterile. The time between collection and the start of the investigation by the microbiological laboratory should not exceed 3 hours.

### 2.10  Biochemical assays for accessory sex organ function

There are various biochemical markers of accessory gland function, e.g., citric acid, zinc, $\gamma$-glutamyl transpeptidase and acid phosphatase for the prostate gland; fructose and prostaglandins for the seminal vesicles; free L-carnitine, glycerophosphocholine, and neutral $\alpha$-glucosidase for the epididymis. An infection can sometimes cause a decrease in the secretion of these markers, but despite this, the total amount of markers present may still be within the normal range. An infection can also cause irreversible damage to the secretory epithelium so that even after treatment the secretion will remain low (Cooper et al., 1990; von der Kammer et al., 1991). The semen of men with ejaculatory duct obstruction or agenesis of the vasa deferentia and seminal vesicles is characterized by low fructose and, in addition, by low volume, low pH, no coagulation, and no characteristic semen odour.

### 2.10.1 Secretory capacity of the prostate

The contents of zinc, citric acid (Gruber & Möllering, 1966) and acid phosphatase (Heite & Wetterauer, 1979) in semen give reliable measures of prostate gland secretion and there are good correlations between these markers. A spectrophotometric assay for zinc is described in Appendix X.

### 2.10.2 Secretory capacity of the seminal vesicles

Fructose in semen reflects the secretory function of the seminal vesicles, and a method for its estimation can be found in Appendix XI.

### 2.10.3 Secretory capacity of the epididymis

L-Carnitine and neutral α-glucosidase are epididymal markers used clinically. There are two isoforms of α-glucosidase in the seminal plasma: the major, neutral one originates solely from the epididymis and the minor, acidic one mainly from the prostate. Neutral α-glucosidase has been shown to be more specific and sensitive for epididymal disorders than L-carnitine and glycerophosphocholine. Its measurement is described in Appendix XII.

## 2.11 Computer-aided sperm analysis

The use of computer-aided sperm analysis (CASA) should provide two advantages over manual methods: (i) high precision and (ii) provision of quantitative data on sperm kinematics. Reliable and repeatable results are possible if appropriate procedures are followed (Davis & Katz, 1992). Many factors are now known to affect the performance of CASA instruments, e.g., sample preparation, frame rate, and sperm concentration (Davis & Katz, 1992; Mortimer, 1994a, b). Guidelines for the use of CASA (Mortimer et al., 1995; European Society of Human Reproduction and Embryology, 1996) should be consulted (see Appendix XIV).

Provided that adequate care is taken in specimen preparation and instrument use, CASA can be used for routine diagnostic applications to monitor the concentration of progressively motile spermatozoa. Strict quality control procedures are necessary to establish and maintain a high standard of instrument operation (see Appendix XIV). Even with quality control and adherence to rigorous procedures, it was previously not feasible to determine sperm concentration by CASA because of difficulties in distinguishing spermatozoa from particulate debris (European Society of Human Reproduction and Embryology, 1996). However, advances in technology, particularly in the use of fluorescent DNA stains with CASA, may now allow sperm concentration to be determined (Zinaman et al., 1996).

Some studies have suggested that CASA estimates of concentration and movement characteristics of progressively motile spermatozoa are significantly related to fertilization rates in vitro and to time to conception (Barratt et al., 1993; Tomlinson et al., 1993; Irvine et al., 1994; Krause, 1995).

## 2.12 Zona-free hamster oocyte test

Sperm–oocyte fusion in the hamster oocyte penetration test is identical to that in the human since fusion with the vitelline membrane of the oocyte is initiated by the plasma membrane overlying the equatorial segment of acrosome-reacted human spermatozoa. The test differs from the physiological situation in that the zona pellucida is absent. A standardized protocol for this test is given in Appendix XV.

The conventional hamster oocyte test depends upon the occurrence of spontaneous acrosome reactions in populations of spermatozoa incubated for prolonged periods of time in vitro. Since this procedure is less efficient than the biological process and may involve different mechanisms, false-negative results (patients whose spermatozoa fail in the hamster oocyte test but which succeed in fertilizing human oocytes in vitro or in vivo) have frequently been recorded (World Health Organization, 1986).

The intracellular signals that initiate the acrosome reaction following sperm–zona pellucida interaction are an influx of calcium and cytoplasmic alkalinization. Both can be generated artificially with the divalent cation ionophore, A23187 (Aitken et al., 1993; Appendix XV).

## 2C RESEARCH TESTS

A wide range of research tests currently under investigation were considered for inclusion in this section. Of these, the following were selected as approaching diagnostic application in the clinic.

## 2.13 Sperm function tests

### 2.13.1 Reactive oxygen species and male infertility

The excessive generation of reactive oxygen species (ROS) and the presence of high concentrations of cytoplasmic enzymes such as creatine phosphokinase may both reflect abnormal or immature spermatozoa with excessively retained cytoplasm in the midpiece (Rao et al., 1989; Gomez et al., 1996).

Reactive oxygen species are metabolites of oxygen and include superoxide anion, hydrogen peroxide, hydroxyl radical, hydroperoxyl radical and nitric oxide. When present in excess, such reactive oxygen species can initiate pathological damage by inducing oxidative damage to cellular lipids, proteins and DNA (Griveau & Le Lannou, 1997). Most cells are equipped with either enzymatic antioxidant systems (superoxide dismutase, glutathione peroxidase and catalase) or nonenzymatic antioxidant systems (uric acid, vitamin C, vitamin E). When these defences are overwhelmed, cell function is affected.

In the human ejaculate, reactive oxygen species are produced by both spermatozoa (Aitken & Clarkson, 1987; Alvarez et al., 1987; Iwasaki & Gagnon, 1992) and leukocytes (Aitken & West, 1990). Seminal plasma possesses antioxidant scavengers and enzymes which may be deficient in some patients (Jones et al., 1979; Smith et al., 1996). The removal of seminal plasma during the preparation of spermatozoa for assisted conception may render these cells vulnerable to oxidative attack. About 40% of men attending infertility clinics and 97% of spinal cord injured men exhibit detectable levels of ROS generation in their semen (Iwasaki & Gagnon, 1992). High ROS production may cause peroxidative damage and loss of sperm function.

Chemiluminescent procedures employing probes such as luminol or lucigenin may be used to measure ROS production (Appendix XVI).

### 2.13.2  Human zona pellucida binding tests

The process of binding of spermatozoa to the zona pellucida leads to initiation of the acrosome reaction, release of lytic acrosomal components and penetration of the spermatozoon through the zona matrix. To evaluate these events, nonviable, nonfertilizable human oocytes from autopsy or surgically removed ovaries or from in vitro fertilization programmes may be used. These oocytes can be kept in high salt solutions for several months (Yanagimachi et al., 1979). One zona pellucida binding assay, termed the hemizona assay (Burkman et al., 1988; Oehninger et al., 1989), involves microdissection of the zona pellucida into equal halves and the exposure of each matching half to the same concentration of test and control spermatozoa. Another sperm–zona binding assay involves differentially labelling the test sample spermatozoa with one fluorescent dye (e.g., fluorescein) and a control sperm sample with another dye (e.g., rhodamine; Liu et al., 1988, 1989). The number of spermatozoa from the test and control samples bound to the same intact zona are counted and reported as a ratio. Both zona binding tests have been shown to be correlated with fertilization rates in vitro. These tests can be performed using salt-stored oocytes (Kruger et al., 1991) but are limited by the availability of human oocytes.

It may be clinically useful to evaluate the number of bound spermatozoa in cases of low or failed in vitro fertilization (Franken et al., 1989; Liu & Baker, 1992). Few or no spermatozoa bound to the zona pellucida usually indicates a sperm defect.

### 2.13.3  Assessment of the acrosome reaction

The assessment of acrosomal status after induction of the acrosome reaction by calcium ionophore (Cummins et al., 1991; Appendix

XVII) identifies acrosome reaction dysfunction (European Society of Human Reproduction and Embryology, 1996). Various staining methods are available for assessing the acrosomal status of human spermatozoa using light or fluorescence microscopy (Cross et al., 1986; De Jonge, 1994; Cross, 1995).

Both microscopy and flow cytometry (Fenichel et al., 1989; Henley et al., 1994) can be used with fluorescent-labelled lectins such as *Pisum sativum* (pea agglutinin) and monoclonal antibodies to examine the acrosome (Cross, 1995). The presence of the outer acrosomal membrane, the acrosomal contents, and the inner acrosomal membrane can be detected by different probes, and the choice of probe influences the time course of detection of acrosome-reacted spermatozoa (Aitken & Brindle, 1993). Viability of the spermatozoa can be determined at the same time with a fluorescent dye (H 33258 bisbenzamine, Hoechst) or by the hypo-osmotic swelling test (see Section 2.8).

The physiological acrosome reaction occurs at the zona pellucida after sperm binding. The development of a valid bioassay for the physiological acrosome reaction of spermatozoa that fertilize oocytes remains difficult, although calcium ionophores or progesterone (Blackmore et al., 1990; Aitken et al., 1996) may be used to assess the competence of capacitated spermatozoa to initiate normal acrosome reactions (see Section 2.12). The clinical relevance of assessments of the induced acrosome reaction remains to be established.

## 2.14 Computer-aided sperm analysis: morphology

Several studies have suggested that assessment of sperm morphology using computerized methods may provide clinically useful information (Katz et al., 1986; Davis & Gravance, 1993; Garrett & Baker, 1995; Garrett et al., 1997; Irvine et al., 1994; Kruger et al., 1995, 1996). Some CASA companies offer packages to examine sperm morphology but few are fully automated and there are problems with the preparation of samples for analysis and with discrimination between spermatozoa and debris. Further development is therefore needed before computer-aided sperm analysis can be recommended for routine assessment of sperm morphology.

# 3 Sperm preparation techniques

The separation of human spermatozoa from seminal plasma to achieve a final preparation with a high percentage of morphologically normal and motile spermatozoa, free from debris and dead spermatozoa, is important for several therapeutic and diagnostic techniques in clinical andrology. Many procedures may be used but there are two main methods of separation (see Appendix XVIII; Mortimer, 1994a, b).

Firstly, spermatozoa may be selected on their ability to swim, known as the 'swim-up' technique. Centrifugation of spermatozoa (including cell debris and leukocytes) prior to swim-up should be avoided because it can result in damage to the sperm membranes, probably by the production of reactive oxygen species (see Section 2.13.1). A direct swim-up from semen is the preferred method for the separation of motile spermatozoa. This technique is performed by layering culture medium over the liquefied semen. Motile spermatozoa then swim into the culture medium (see Appendix XVIII.2).

The second method of selecting spermatozoa is by the use of density gradients. A simple two-step preparation is the most extensively used of such methods (Appendix XVIII.3). In general, the direct swim-up technique is used when the semen samples are considered to be normal. For semen with suboptimal characteristics, alternative preparations are generally preferred.

It may be necessary to select the sperm preparation technique according to the individual semen samples (see Canale et al., 1994; Smith et al., 1996). The efficiency of the various techniques is usually expressed as the absolute number or the relative yield of morphologically normal motile spermatozoa. In some cases, the functional capacity of the prepared spermatozoa may be determined in, for example, the zona-free hamster oocyte test (Appendix XV) to identify the most suitable method of preparation.

In the past, clinical studies have concentrated on the advantages and disadvantages of using Percoll. However, Percoll was recently withdrawn for the separation of spermatozoa for use in human clinical applications and now may be used only for research purposes. Instead, other methods are becoming available. One is the use of preparations of colloidal silica coated with silane. Another is the use of density gradients (Gellert-Mortimer et al., 1988; Sbracia et al., 1996; see Appendix XVIII). In addition, glass wool columns are reported to be as effective as Percoll gradients were for the separation of spermatozoa from semen with suboptimal characteristics (Rhemrev et al., 1989; Johnson et al., 1996).

# 4 Quality control in the andrology laboratory

## 4.1 Introduction

Quality control (QC) of semen analysis is essential for the detection and correction of systematic errors and high variability. Regular QC assessment by the laboratory supervisor is required for laboratory accreditation and to maintain accuracy, precision and competence in the andrology laboratory. QC activities performed within one laboratory are referred to as internal quality control (IQC). External quality assessment (EQA) is the evaluation of results for the same samples in several laboratories. Quality assurance is a wider concept including optimization of the services provided.

The management of QC procedures requires an understanding of the source and magnitude of measurement errors. Semen analysis is subject to relatively large random errors associated with counting limited numbers of spermatozoa. The large disagreements found between the assessments of sperm concentration and morphology by different laboratories (Neuwinger et al., 1990; Matson, 1995) underlines the need for improved QC and standardization. Until there are universally accepted standard methods and definitions of motility and morphology, it will not be possible to compare results from different laboratories. Results from each laboratory will need to be interpreted against that laboratory's own reference ranges.

Several publications deal with QC in the andrology laboratory (Mortimer et al., 1986, 1989; Dunphy et al., 1989; Knuth et al., 1989; Cooper et al., 1992; Mortimer, 1994a, b; Clements et al., 1995). The statistical aspects of QC are found in some textbooks and statistical packages (Barnett, 1979). A practical approach to QC for an andrology laboratory is outlined in this chapter.

## 4.2 Nature of errors in measurement

Any measurement has a degree of error, the magnitude of which is described by a confidence interval with an upper and a lower limit. A precise measurement is one in which the limits lie close together, and the result is accurate when there is minimum departure from the true value. There are two classes of error: 'random' and 'systematic'. Random errors, causing lack of precision, arise from chance differences in readings or sampling; they can be assessed by repeated measurements by the same observer and equipment. Systematic errors (sometimes referred to as 'bias') are more insidious since they arise from factors that alter the result in one direction only and thus create departures that cannot be detected by repeated measurements. QC procedures are required to detect and assess both random and systematic errors in routine semen analysis.

4.2.1   *Statistical counting errors in semen analysis*
The random distribution of spermatozoa, even when the sample is well mixed, accounts for most of the variability or lack of precision in semen analysis results. The measurement of sperm concentration, motility and morphology all involve counting a limited number of spermatozoa presumed to be representative of the whole sample. The sampling variation created by selecting either a fixed volume for estimating concentration or a fixed number of spermatozoa for classifying motility or morphology is a random error commonly referred to as the (statistical) counting error. The relative magnitude of the counting error is inversely related to the square root of the number of spermatozoa assessed. Knowledge of counting error is crucial for assessing the precision of semen analysis and for implementing QC procedures to identify other sources of error.

*Counting errors in measurement of sperm concentration*
To measure sperm concentration, the spermatozoa in a fixed volume of diluted semen are counted in a haemocytometer. If randomly distributed throughout the chamber, the exact number of spermatozoa in a given volume follows the Poisson distribution, whose variance is equal to the number counted. Thus, when $N$ spermatozoa are counted, the sampling variance is $N$, the standard error is $\sqrt{N}$, and the percentage error $100\sqrt{N}/N$. The 95% confidence interval for the number of spermatozoa in the volume of semen is approximately $N \pm 1.96 \sqrt{N}$. Therefore, if 100 spermatozoa are counted, the standard error of the count is 10 (10%) and the 95% confidence interval for the number of spermatozoa in the volume of semen counted is 80–120. Similarly, if 200 spermatozoa are counted, the standard error is 14 (7%) with a 95% confidence interval of 172–228. To achieve a precision represented by a percentage error of 2.5% it is necessary to count 1600 spermatozoa.

*Counting errors in measurement of sperm motility and morphology*
When spermatozoa are classified into two or more classes (such as 'normal' or 'abnormal' morphology, 'progressive' or 'nonprogressive' motility) the standard error of the estimated percentage ($p$) within a class depends on the true, but unknown percentage as well as on the number of spermatozoa counted ($N$). The estimated standard error is

$\sqrt{p(100-p)/N}$. Thus if 100 spermatozoa are counted and the true percentage with normal morphology is 20%, the standard error of the estimated percentage of normal spermatozoa is 4.0%. The corresponding 95% confidence interval is 12.2%–27.8%. If 200 spermatozoa are counted, the standard error becomes 2.8% with a 95% confidence interval of 14.5%–25.5%. If 400 spermatozoa are counted, the standard error is further reduced to 2.0% with a 95% confidence interval of 16.1%–23.9%.

*Minimizing statistical counting error*
While counting error can be reduced by assessing greater numbers of spermatozoa, a balance must be struck between the gain in statistical precision and the possible loss of accuracy in the technician's work due to fatigue.

4.2.2 *Other errors in semen analysis*
Repeated analyses by the same technician and procedure will yield greater variability than the counting error alone, because additional random errors are usually present. These may arise from inadequate mixing (common with viscous and agglutinated samples), technician stress (erratic counting or recording error), poor technique (e.g., careless pipetting or handling during slide or chamber preparation), or instrument variation (e.g., worn automatic pipettes, which may reduce reproducibility during sampling and dilution). In contrast, results with less variability than the expected counting error suggest the possibility of recording errors or of bias induced by knowledge of previous measurements.

Measurements repeated by different technicians may differ because of systematic differences, or biases from consistent calculation errors, or differences in the classification of morphology and motility. For example, the percentage of motile spermatozoa is commonly overestimated because the eye is attracted to movement. This error can be reduced by systematically counting all motile spermatozoa first and then counting the immotile spermatozoa in the same area.

4.2.3 *The importance of quality control*
The precision or reproducibility of a semen analysis can be assessed from the results of repeated measurements of the same sample, a method which, together with regular calibration of equipment, forms the basis of IQC. Intratechnician precision is determined from the replicate estimates or repeated analyses of the same masked sample. Intertechnician intralaboratory precision is determined by independent analyses of the same sample. Interlaboratory variability is evaluated by EQA. IQC should ensure that optimal precision is maintained in the andrology laboratory and that there is no gradual shift in stan-

dards. IQC is essential both when a single technician makes infrequent assessments or several technicians work together. EQA is essential to ensure that different laboratories produce comparable results and can indicate when a laboratory's methods should be adjusted.

### 4.3 Practical approaches to quality control

The QC procedures described below are the minimum that should be implemented in an andrology laboratory. The QC procedures for other aspects of good laboratory practice, such as maintaining a constant temperature in incubators and calibrating balances, are assumed to be routinely conducted.

At all times – surveillance and correlation of results within samples.

Weekly – analysis of replicate measurements of the main semen variables by different technicians.

Monthly – analysis of mean results of tests.

Quarterly – participation in an EQA scheme, calibration of pipettes.

Yearly – calibration of counting chambers and other equipment (see Appendix XIX).

The QC activity in a laboratory will vary depending on the work load and experience of the technicians. In busy laboratories between 1% and 5% of samples should be for IQC. It is important for the QC samples to be masked, and they should be analysed as part of routine laboratory work. In this way IQC will help to maintain accuracy and precision in routine semen analysis.

#### 4.3.1 Routine surveillance and correlation of results within samples

Results must be checked for errors of transcription and patient identification. Unusual results that do not match other aspects of the semen analysis may suggest such errors. Estimates of sperm concentration, motility, and morphology from the initial microscopic examination of the undiluted semen can be used as a rough check on the final result. The percentage of live and motile spermatozoa should be consistent. Alarm results are unusual occurrences requiring urgent attention. Examples of alarm results for the laboratory include zero or unexpected loss of sperm motility, which may be caused by temperature change or contamination with sperm toxins. Alarm results for the clinician include a patient who previously had spermatozoa in the semen becoming azoospermic or being unable to produce a sample.

For sperm concentration, independent duplicate counts in the two parts of the counting chamber are compared (see Section 2.5.2, Fig. 2.6). The difference between independent counts on equal volumes from the same sample is expected to be zero, with standard error equal to the square root of the sum of the two counts. In about 95% of duplicate samples the difference between the two counts will be less than 1.96 standard errors. If not, a systematic error is suspected and the sample is remixed, diluted again and the procedure repeated. In about 5% of samples, differences greater than 1.96 standard errors will occur as a result of chance variation alone, and the count will have been repeated unnecessarily. However, this small additional work is an assurance that there have been no systematic errors.

Similar procedures are followed for duplicate estimates of the percentages of spermatozoa with different motility grades (Section 2.4.3, Fig. 2.3) and morphological characteristics (Section 2.5.4). Two independent estimates, $p_1$ and $p_2$, are made on $N$ spermatozoa in each sample and compared. The limit of expected difference $d$ is given by $d = |p_1 - p_2| < 1.96\sqrt{2\bar{p}(100-\bar{p})/N}$ where $\bar{p} = (p_1 + p_2)/2$ is the average percentage. Using these limits, 5% of duplicates will be rejected from chance variation alone.

### 4.3.2 Weekly internal quality control: assessing intra- and inter-technician variability

A simple method of IQC involves replicate measurements performed on separate aliquots of the sample and carried through all stages of the analysis. Assessing the slide or chamber twice on the same occasion is not true replication. It does not assess errors of preparation or dilution. The replicate assessments should be performed in the same way as routine samples with technicians unaware that IQC samples are being assessed. IQC should include assessments of sperm concentration, sperm motility grades, sperm morphology, the immunobead test, the mixed agglutination reaction, and any other results reported by the laboratory. Stored semen samples (see Appendix XIX) can be used for IQC and have the advantage that the true or target value is known, or can be estimated. An easier approach is for the same fresh sample, or pool of several samples, to be analysed independently by different technicians, which will enable the variability between these technicians to be assessed; however, the true value is not known and thus systematic error or bias of the group cannot be estimated. The IQC of sperm motility presents special problems since motility may decline over time and thus needs to be assessed first and at about the same time by all the technicians.

The statistical procedures for analysing and reporting the IQC results are presented below. Some of these procedures depend on the true or target value being known (or estimated from the first ten or so determinations). Statistical packages for laboratory QC are available and can be used for analysis and the presentation of results. The procedures are easier to interpret and compute if the same number of technicians participate in each QC determination. If this is not possible, one or more of the technicians can assess the sample a second time so that the number of determinations on each QC sample is the same. Some computer programmes can accommodate a variable number of observers.

Table 4.1. *Factors for determining control limits for $X_{bar}$ and S charts based on the average standard deviation ($S_{bar}$)*

| Number of technicians ($n$) | SD estimate ($c_n$) | $X_{bar}$ chart control limits | | S chart control limits | | | |
|---|---|---|---|---|---|---|---|
| | | Warning ($A_2$) | Action ($A_3$) | Lower action ($s_{0.999}$) | Lower warning ($s_{0.975}$) | Upper warning ($s_{0.025}$) | Upper action ($s_{0.001}$) |
| 2 | 1.253 | 1.772 | 2.659 | 0.002 | 0.039 | 2.809 | 4.124 |
| 3 | 1.128 | 1.303 | 1.954 | 0.036 | 0.180 | 2.167 | 2.966 |
| 4 | 1.085 | 1.085 | 1.628 | 0.098 | 0.291 | 1.916 | 2.527 |
| 5 | 1.064 | 0.952 | 1.427 | 0.160 | 0.370 | 1.776 | 2.286 |
| 6 | 1.051 | 0.858 | 1.287 | 0.215 | 0.428 | 1.684 | 2.129 |
| 7 | 1.042 | 0.788 | 1.182 | 0.263 | 0.473 | 1.618 | 2.017 |
| 8 | 1.036 | 0.733 | 1.099 | 0.303 | 0.509 | 1.567 | 1.932 |
| 9 | 1.032 | 0.688 | 1.032 | 0.338 | 0.539 | 1.527 | 1.864 |
| 10 | 1.028 | 0.650 | 0.975 | 0.368 | 0.563 | 1.495 | 1.809 |

*IQC with stored samples: sperm concentration*

The results obtained by each technician on the QC sample are tabulated and plotted on a graph against the sample (or week) number. The mean and standard deviation of the results on each sample are computed and also plotted against the sample (or week) number on $X_{bar}$ and S control charts, which are used to determine whether the results obtained on the new QC sample differ from the previous determinations or whether the differences between technicians are greater than would be expected as a result of random variation alone.

When at least five, preferably ten, QC samples have been analysed, the average of the means ($X_{bar}$) and standard deviations ($S_{bar}$) are used to establish control limits on the $X_{bar}$ chart at 2 and 3 standard errors (warning and action control limits) either side of the target value. These are given by $X_{bar} \pm A_{2,n} \times S_{bar}$ and $X_{bar} \pm A_{3,n} \times S_{bar}$, where the values of the coefficients $A_{2,n}$ and $A_{3,n}$ are read from Table 4.1 for the corresponding number of technicians ($n$). The control limits are used to monitor the results obtained on future QC samples. An alternative is to compute the control limits directly as $X_{bar} \pm 2s/\sqrt{n}$ and $X_{bar} \pm 3s/\sqrt{n}$ from the pooled between-technician standard deviation ($s$). This pooled standard deviation is greater than the average of the sample standard deviations $S_{bar}$ and can be computed directly or obtained by multiplying $S_{bar}$ by the factor $c_n$ (Table 4.1). This factor is the amount by which the average standard deviation underestimates the pooled standard deviation in samples of size $n$ from a normal distribution. A worked example is given in Box 4.1.

**Box 4.1: Determining control limits for the $X_{bar}$ chart**

The table below shows the sperm concentrations measured by each of four technicians on the first ten QC samples and the calculation of the mean and the standard deviation of each sample.

*Sperm concentration (million/ml)*

| Sample | 1 | 2 | 3 | 4 | 5 | 6 | 7 | 8 | 9 | 10 |
|---|---|---|---|---|---|---|---|---|---|---|
| Technician A | 38 | 35 | 40 | 34 | 38 | 36 | 44 | 43 | 39 | 43 |
| Technician B | 42 | 36 | 42 | 40 | 40 | 40 | 43 | 43 | 46 | 40 |
| Technician C | 38 | 43 | 40 | 51 | 38 | 33 | 39 | 45 | 35 | 39 |
| Technician D | 34 | 36 | 36 | 37 | 36 | 39 | 42 | 43 | 46 | 34 |
| Mean | 38.0 | 37.5 | 39.5 | 40.5 | 38.0 | 37.0 | 42.0 | 43.5 | 41.5 | 39.0 |
| SD | 3.27 | 3.70 | 2.52 | 7.42 | 1.63 | 3.16 | 2.16 | 1.00 | 5.45 | 3.74 |

For the first ten QC samples the average of the means ($X_{bar}$) is:

$$(38.0 + 37.5 + ... + 39.0)/10 = 39.7,$$

and the average of the standard deviations ($S_{bar}$) is:

$$(3.27 + 3.70 + ... + 3.74)/10 = 3.40.$$

The values of the coefficients $A_{2,n}$ and $A_{3,n}$ in Table 4.1 for samples of size $n = 4$ are 1.085 and 1.628, respectively. Thus the inner (warning) control limits (two standard errors from the mean) are given by:

$$X_{bar} \pm A_{2,n} \times S_{bar} = 39.7 \pm 1.085 \times 3.40 \text{ or } 36.0 \text{ and } 43.3 \text{ million/ml.}$$

Similarly the outer (action) control limits are given by:

$$X_{bar} \pm A_{3,n} \times S_{bar} = 39.7 \pm 1.628 \times 3.40 \text{ or } 34.1 \text{ and } 45.2 \text{ million/ml.}$$

These control limits are added to the $X_{bar}$ chart (Fig. 4.1) to monitor the results of future QC samples.

Fig. 4.1. $X_{bar}$ chart

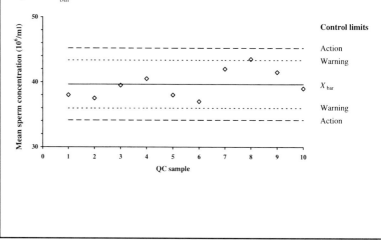

Table 4.2. *Basic control rules for QC chart*

| Control rule | Error sensitivity |
| --- | --- |
| One result outside action limits | Random or systematic error |
| Two consecutive results *both* above the upper warning limit or *both* below the lower warning limit | Systematic error |
| Two consecutive results, one above the upper and one below the lower warning limit | Random error |
| Eight consecutive results *all above* or *all below* the mean | Systematic error |

There are basic control rules to monitor performance of future QC assessments on the QC chart (Table 4.2). If the QC sample is 'rejected', the sensitivity of the alarm to the different types of error (random or systematic) should direct the investigation into possible causes. Systematic error is also suspected if there is a succession of seven points that are either all falling or all rising.

The $X_{bar}$ chart is mainly designed to detect changes from the target value, or an overall increase in variability. It is less sensitive in detecting whether technicians are producing highly variable results or systematically under- or overestimating. For this purpose, the range of values on each QC sample can be monitored on an $R_{bar}$ chart in a similar way to the $X_{bar}$ chart, with warning and action limits set accordingly. A similar chart with more sensitivity is the $S$ chart, based on the sample standard deviations. Since the distribution of the standard deviation is not symmetrical, the warning and action limits are chosen in such a way that the probability of a new observation falling outside the control limits is the same as for the $X_{bar}$ chart if there are no changes in accuracy or precision. Thus the warning and action limits will be crossed in 5% and 0.2% of future samples as a result of random variation alone. These limits are determined from the $\chi^2$ distribution, and the factors $s_{\alpha,n}$ required to multiply the average standard deviation $S_{bar}$ are given in Table 4.1. A worked example is given in Box 4.2. Similar rules to those in Table 4.2 for monitoring performance on future QC samples are applied to the $S$ chart. Results that fall below the lower limits on the $S$ chart suggest unexpectedly small variation, which may indicate a genuine improvement in the level of agreement between technicians, or possible collusion.

The estimates of the mean and the standard deviation can be recomputed after every 10 samples and the control limits updated using the new values for $X_{bar}$ and $S_{bar}$ provided there have been no problems with QC. Before the QC samples run out, a new pool should be prepared and the first 10 samples of the new batch analysed together with the remaining samples of the old batch to establish the new control limits.

### Assessing systematic differences between technicians

The consistency of results between technicians within the laboratory is an important aspect of IQC. However, some technicians may systematically over- or under-estimate the sperm concentration. This should be assessed after every group of 5 or 10 QC samples by two-way analysis of variance with factors for QC samples and technicians (see below). Since the QC samples are all from the same stored pool, significant differences between samples are not expected, and significant differences between technicians would suggest systematic bias in the assessment by one or more technicians.

### IQC with stored samples: sperm motility and morphology

The QC procedures for the assessment of sperm motility and morphology follow the same steps as those outlined above for sperm concentration, except that percentages are being assessed. Since the total number of spermatozoa counted is large, the limits for the control charts can be set using the normal distribution. The approximation is adequate for percentages that lie in the range 20% to 80%, but less good if the percentages are low (<10%) or high (>90%).

For sperm morphology, many slides can be made from a single semen sample. These slides can be prepared from samples with good, medium, or poor quality spermatozoa and one slide from each introduced into the QC assessment. The slides must be masked to prevent recognition as QC samples. The slides can be reused and new ones prepared once they deteriorate. Video tapes can be used for motility QC assessment.

The same basic principles for IQC described above are followed. Once a series of QC determinations has been made, the $X_{bar}$ and $S$ charts can be constructed and warning and action limits set. The standard deviation of the estimated percentage $p$ is $\sqrt{p(100-p)/N}$,

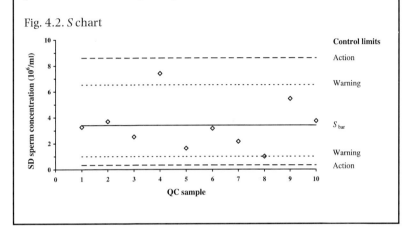
where $N$ is the number of spermatozoa classified. For values of $p$ in the range 20% to 80% and a total of 400 spermatozoa classified, the standard deviation lies in the range 2.0% to 2.5%, with the maximum value when $p$ is 50%. The standard deviation of individual readings should be close to these values. However, the average standard deviation $S_{bar}$ will be greater than 2.5% as a result of the additional variation between technicians, and reducing $S_{bar}$ to the theoretical minimum will be the goal. Only experienced technicians who have achieved a high degree of consistency and standardization will be able to reach this limit. If performance is close to the theoretical limit, then the warning and action limits on the $X_{bar}$ and S control charts can be set using the theoretical standard deviation in preference to the observed standard deviation $S_{bar}$.

If the QC samples have percentages less than 20% or greater than 80%, then a modification to the above procedure may give more appropriate control limits. The angular (or arc sin square root) transformation $z = \sin^{-1}\sqrt{p/100}$ has the property that the standard deviation of $z$ is given by $1/(2\sqrt{N})$ radians and depends only on the number of spermatozoa counted, $N$, and not on the true percentage. This means that the probability of crossing the warning and action limits as a result of random variation alone is closer to the theoretical level. For sperm motility or morphology based on classifying 400 spermatozoa, the standard deviation of $z$ is 0.025 radians, which corresponds to the lowest theoretical limit.

As with the QC of sperm concentration, the two-way analysis of variance is an important step in identifying any consistent under- or over-estimation by certain technicians and in identifying ways in which quality and consistency can be improved.

*IQC with fresh samples: sperm concentration, motility and morphology*
The QC procedures based on the assessment of fresh semen samples are similar to those described above for the stored sample, with the exception that the $X_{bar}$ chart cannot be used as there is no target mean value. However, the primary QC procedures are the $S$ chart for assessing variability between technicians, which is plotted after each QC sample, and the two-way analysis of variance for assessing systematic differences between technicians after every five or ten QC samples.

The two-way analysis of variance is described in many statistical textbooks (for example, Altman, 1991) and is available in packages for computers, together with statistical tests for the significance of differences between technicians. The worked example (Box 4.3) illustrates how to compute the standard error of the differences between technicians directly and assess whether these are greater than would be expected from chance variation alone. When performing computations directly from the observations, a sufficient number of decimal places must be kept to avoid any rounding errors. A formal statistical test for differences between technicians is based on the $F$-test from the two-way analysis of variance table, which can be obtained directly from most statistical computer programs. The error root mean square ($\hat{\sigma}$) is the square root of the residual, or error, mean square from the analysis of variance table. Mean differences greater than about 2.5 standard errors are unlikely to result from chance variation alone. Whether the differences between technicians are significant or not, it is necessary to review the technicians' means or mean differences to identify which are greater than expected. Not all computer packages provide the standard error of the differences between technicians, $se(m_j)$, which may have to be computed separately. Substantial differences between technicians should prompt a review of all procedures to discover ways in which their consistency can be improved.

## 4.4  Monitoring monthly means

While the primary IQC procedures are based on the assessment of differences between and within technicians, useful additional information can be obtained from monitoring trends in semen analysis results from patients. The mean values of each variable for all the patients examined over a certain period (e.g., monthly) can be plotted

**Box 4.3: Assessing systematic differences between technicians**

The table below shows sperm concentrations estimated by each of three technicians on five QC samples.

*Sperm concentration (million/ml)*

| Sample | 1 | 2 | 3 | 4 | 5 |
|---|---|---|---|---|---|
| Technician A | 108 | 45 | 100 | 50 | 92 |
| Technician B | 103 | 47 | 102 | 50 | 96 |
| Technician C | 104 | 46 | 89 | 41 | 88 |
| Sample mean | 105.0 | 46.0 | 97.0 | 47.0 | 92.0 |

The differences from the sample mean ($d_{ij}$) are computed by subtracting the semen sample mean from each observation:

*Differences ($d_{ij}$) from sample mean (million/ml)*

| Sample | 1 | 2 | 3 | 4 | 5 |
|---|---|---|---|---|---|
| Technician A | 3.0 | −1.0 | 3.0 | 3.0 | 0.0 |
| Technician B | −2.0 | 1.0 | 5.0 | 3.0 | 4.0 |
| Technician C | −1.0 | 0.0 | −8.0 | −6.0 | −4.0 |

The mean, $m_j = \sum_i d_{ij}/n$, and standard deviation, $s_j = \sqrt{\sum_i d_{ij}^2/(n-1)}$, of these differences are computed for each technician, where $n$ is the number of semen samples.

*Mean and standard deviation of differences (million/ml)*

| | Mean $(m_j)$ | SD $(s_j)$ | Mean/standard error $(m_j/se(m_j))$ |
|---|---|---|---|
| Technician A | 1.600 | 1.949 | 1.301 |
| Technician B | 2.200 | 2.775 | 1.788 |
| Technician C | −3.800 | 3.347 | −3.089 |

Technician C's mean difference is 3.8 million/ml below the mean of each QC sample, or 5.7 $(=-3.8-[1.6+2.2]/2)$ million/ml less than the average of the other two technicians. To assess whether the degree of underestimation is compatible with chance variation, the error root mean square, $\hat{\sigma} = \sqrt{\sum_j s_j^2/(t-1)}$, where $t$ is the number of technicians, is computed from the standard deviations of the technicians' differences. In this example it is 3.369 million/ml. The standard error of each technician's mean difference is given by $se(m_j) = \hat{\sigma}\sqrt{(1-1/t)/n}$ and is 1.230 million/ml. The absolute value of Technician C's mean difference (3.8 million/ml) is greater than 3 standard errors and is significantly different from the expected value of zero if there are no systematic differences between the technicians.

A formal statistical test of differences between technicians is based on the F-test from the two-way analysis of variance with factors for technicians and QC samples. The analysis of variance table, using the above sperm concentrations, is given below.

*Two-way analysis of variance*

| Source | Sum of squares | Degrees of freedom | Mean square | F-ratio | P-value |
|---|---|---|---|---|---|
| QC samples | 9807.6 | 4 | 2451.90 | 216.03 | <0.001 |
| Technicians | 109.2 | 2 | 54.60 | 4.81 | 0.042 |
| Error | 90.8 | 8 | 11.35 | | |
| Total | 10007.6 | 14 | | | |

The error root mean square is $\sqrt{11.35} = 3.369$ million/ml, the same as that obtained above. As expected, the differences between QC samples are very large ($P<0.001$) since they are taken from different fresh semen samples. The F-test for differences between technicians ($F=4.81$ with 2 and 8 degrees of freedom, $P=0.042$) is significant at the 0.05 level and suggests that these differences are greater than would be expected from random variation alone.

on an $X_{bar}$ chart with warning and action limits 2 and 3 standard errors either side of the mean. The standard error is estimated from the standard deviation of the original observations divided by the square root of the number of semen analyses in each interval, or directly from the observed distribution of the mean (see Box 4.4). The control limits should be determined using at least 6 months' observations and revised regularly. There should be at least 20 results for each mean, and a small laboratory may have to pool results from more than one month. Deviations outside the control limits may indicate uncontrolled changes in laboratory practice or shifting trends in assessment, provided that the patient characteristics did not change markedly over the period studied (see Knuth et al., 1989). Refinements to the method include monitoring monthly means of patients with normal values and the use of cumulative sum (CUSUM) charts (Barnett, 1979) for the rapid detection of any systematic departures from the mean.

## 4.5 Response to results outside control limits

The results of QC must be reviewed regularly by the laboratory supervisor, and the report must be signed and dated. When results outside control limits appear, the probable cause and action taken should also be recorded. If the problem is not obvious, the QC samples should be reanalysed to check if the first result was unusual. If the QC result remains outside control limits when repeated, the analysis of routine

The following properties may be ascribed to the cervix and its secretions: (a) receptivity to sperm penetration at, or near, ovulation and interference with penetration at other times, (b) protection of spermatozoa from the hostile environment of the vagina and from being phagocytosed, (c) supplementation of the energy requirements of spermatozoa, (d) filtration (i.e., sperm selection on the basis of differential motility and morphology), (e) provision of a short-term sperm reservoir, and (f) initiation of sperm capacitation.

Spermatozoa within the mucus are, at all times, suspended in a fluid medium. The interaction of spermatozoa with the secretions of the female reproductive tract is of critical importance for the survival and functional ability of spermatozoa. There is no practical method at present of evaluating the effects of human uterine and tubal fluids on spermatozoa, but cervical mucus is readily available for sampling and study. Evaluation of sperm–cervical mucus interaction therefore, is an important measure to be included in any complete investigation of infertility. A finding of abnormal sperm–cervical mucus interaction may be an indication for artificial insemination or other forms of assisted reproduction.

## 5.2 Collection and preservation of cervical mucus

### 5.2.1 Collection procedure
The cervix is exposed with a speculum and the external os is gently wiped with a cotton swab to remove the external pool of vaginal contaminants. The exocervical mucus is removed with the swab or with forceps. Cervical mucus is collected from the endocervical canal by any one of the following methods. The mucus can be aspirated with a tuberculin syringe (without a needle), a mucus syringe, a pipette, or a polyethylene tube. Whenever possible, the quality of the mucus should be evaluated immediately on collection. If this is not possible, the mucus should be preserved (Section 5.2.2) until it can be tested.

When mucus is collected by aspiration, it is important to standardize the manner in which suction pressure is applied to the collection device (syringe, catheter, etc.). Suction is initiated after the tip of the device has been advanced approximately 1 cm into the cervical canal. Suction is then maintained as the device is withdrawn. Just prior to withdrawal of the device from the external cervical os, suction pressure is released. It is then advisable to clamp the catheter to protect against accumulation of air bubbles or vaginal material in the collected mucus when the device is removed from the cervical canal.

When cervical mucus is to be collected at a time other than at mid-cycle, its production can be increased by the administration of 20 to 80 µg/day ethinyloestradiol, beginning, e.g., on the fifth day of a given cycle for a period of up to 10 days. The mucus may be collected within the period 7–10 days after the start of administration of ethinyloestradiol. This procedure will produce a more hydrated, and therefore less viscous, mucus secretion (Eggert-Kruse et al., 1989). While this approach may be useful in assessing sperm–mucus interaction in vitro, it will not necessarily reflect the in vivo situation for the couple when hormones are not administered.

### 5.2.2 *Storage and preservation*

Mucus can be preserved either in the original tuberculin syringe or polyethylene tube or in small test tubes and sealed with a stopper or with paraffin paper to avoid dehydration. Care should be taken to minimize the air space in the storage container. The samples should be preserved in a refrigerator at 4 °C for a period not exceeding 5 days. If possible, mucus specimens should be utilized within 2 days of collection, and the interval between collection and use should always be noted. Rheological and sperm penetration tests should not be performed on mucus specimens that have been frozen and thawed.

## 5.3 Evaluation of cervical mucus

Evaluation of the properties of cervical mucus includes assessment of spinnbarkeit, ferning (crystallization), consistency and pH. Appendix XX gives a sample form for recording the postcoital test in which these cervical mucus properties are scored according to the system devised by Moghissi (1976), based on the original proposal of Insler et al. (1972). The maximum score is 15. A score greater than 10 is usually indicative of a good cervical mucus favouring sperm penetration, and a score less than 10 may represent unfavourable cervical mucus. The score is derived from the volume of cervical mucus collected (Section 5.3.1) and four variables (Sections 5.3.2 to 5.3.5) describing its characteristics and appearance. The pH of the mucus is not included in the total cervical mucus score, but should be measured as an important determinant of sperm–mucus interaction (Eggert-Kruse et al., 1993).

### 5.3.1 *Volume*

Volume is scored as follows:
0 = 0 ml,
1 = 0.1 ml,
2 = 0.2 ml,
3 = 0.3 ml or more.

### 5.3.2 *Consistency*

The consistency of cervical mucus is the most important factor influencing sperm penetration. There is little resistance to sperm migration through the cervical mucus in mid-cycle, but viscous mucus such as that observed during the luteal phase forms a more formidable barrier. Cellular debris and leukocytes in cervical mucus impede sperm migration. Gross endocervicitis has been alleged to be associated with reduced fertility.

Consistency is scored as follows:

0 = thick, highly viscous, premenstrual mucus,
1 = mucus of intermediate viscosity,
2 = mildly viscous mucus,
3 = watery, minimally viscous, mid-cycle (preovulatory) mucus.

### 5.3.3 Ferning

Ferning (Fig. 5.1) is scored by examination of cervical mucus which is air-dried on glass microscope slides. Such preparations reveal various patterns of crystallization which may have a fern-like appearance. Depending on the composition of the mucus the 'ferns' may have only a primary stem or the stem may branch once, twice or three times to produce secondary, tertiary and quaternary stems, respectively. Several fields around the preparation are observed and the score is expressed as the highest degree of ferning that is *typical* of the specimen according to the following definitions:

0 = no crystallization,
1 = atypical fern formation,
2 = primary and secondary stem ferning,
3 = tertiary and quarternary stem ferning.

### 5.3.4 Spinnbarkeit

The cervical mucus on a microscope slide is touched with a cover slip, or a second slide held crosswise, which is lifted gently. The length of the cervical mucus thread stretched in between is estimated in centimetres and is scored as follows:

0 = <1 cm,
1 = 1–4 cm,
2 = 5–8 cm,
3 = 9 cm or more.

### 5.3.5 Cellularity

It is recommended that all cell counts be expressed in cells/mm$^3$ (i.e., per $\mu$l). An estimate of the number of leukocytes and other cells in the cervical mucus is traditionally based on the number counted per high-power microscope field or HPF. One combination of microscope optics to produce the HPF is a 10× wide-field ocular lens (aperture size 20 mm) and a 40× objective lens. Because the diameter of the microscope field is equal to the diameter of the the aperture of the ocular lens divided by the magnification of the objective lens, these optics result in a microscope field with a diameter of approximately 500 $\mu$m. The depth of the preparation can also be standardized by supporting the coverslip on silicone grease containing 100 μm glass beads (Drobnis et al., 1988). If the field is 100 μm deep, its volume must be 0.02 mm³. Thus, a count of 10 cells/HPF is equivalent to approximately 500 cells/mm³ under these conditions.

The rank scores for cells are:

$0 = > 20$ cells/HPF or $>1000$ cells/mm³
$1 = 11–20$ cells/HPF or $501–1000$ cells/mm³
$2 = 1–10$ cells/HPF or $1–500$ cells/mm³
$3 = 0$ cells

### 5.3.6 pH

The pH of cervical mucus from the endocervical canal should be obtained with pH paper, range 6.4–8.0, *in situ* or immediately following collection. If the pH is measured *in situ*, care should be taken to measure it correctly, since the pH of exocervical mucus is always lower than that of mucus in the endocervical canal. Care should also be taken to avoid contamination with secretions of the vagina, which have an acidic pH.

Spermatozoa are susceptible to changes in pH of the cervical mucus. Acid mucus immobilizes spermatozoa, whereas alkaline mucus may enhance motility. Excessive alkalinity of the cervical mucus (pH greater than 8.5) may, however, adversely affect the viability of spermatozoa. The optimum pH value for sperm migration and survival in the cervical mucus is between 7.0 and 8.5, which represents the pH range of normal, mid-cycle cervical mucus. However, a pH value between 6.0 and 7.0 may still be compatible with sperm penetration.

In some cases cervical mucus may be substantially more acidic. This can be due either to abnormal secretion or to the presence of a bacterial infection.

## 5.4 Interaction between sperm and cervical mucus

Cervical mucus is receptive to sperm migration for a limited time during the cycle. Oestrogen-influenced mucus favours penetration. The length of time during which spermatozoa can penetrate cervical mucus varies considerably from one woman to another, and may vary in the same individual from one cycle to another. Abnormality of sperm–cervical mucus interaction should not be inferred without repeated tests in separate cycles.

### 5.4.1 In vivo (postcoital) test

(i) *Timing*  Postcoital tests should be performed prior to ovulation and as closely as possible to the time of ovulation as determined by clinical criteria, i.e., usual cycle length, basal body temperature, cervical mucus changes, vaginal cytology, and, when available, serum or urinary oestrogen assays and an ovarian ultrasound examination. It is important for all laboratories to evaluate the mucus at a standard time after coitus. This time should be from 9 to 24 hours.

(ii) *Suggested instructions to patients in preparation for the postcoital test*

(a) You and your partner should abstain from intercourse for at least 2 days before the test.

(b) The most suitable day for your test is (day) (month) (year). Intercourse should take place the night before this day according to your normal practice.

(c) Do not use any vaginal lubricants during intercourse and do not douche after intercourse. You may take a shower after intercourse but do not take a full bath.

(d) Report to the clinic for the test at (time), on (day) (month) (year).

(iii) *Technique of postcoital test*  A nonlubricated speculum is inserted into the vagina and a sample of the fluid pool in the posterior vaginal fornix is aspirated with a tuberculin syringe (without needle), a pipette, or a polyethylene tube. Using a different syringe or catheter, a sample of mucus is then aspirated from the endocervical canal (Section 5.2.1), placed on a glass microscope slide, covered with a cover slip, and examined at a standard depth under a phase-contrast microscope (Section 5.3.5).

(iv) *Vaginal pool sample*  Spermatozoa are usually killed in the vagina within two hours. The vaginal pool sample is examined to ensure that semen has been deposited in the vagina.

(v) *Cervical mucus sample*  The number of spermatozoa in the lower part of the cervical canal varies with time elapsed after intercourse. Some 2–3 hours after coitus, there is a large accumulation of spermatozoa in the lower part of the cervical canal.

It is recommended that the concentration of spermatozoa within the mucus be expressed in standard units (number of spermatozoa/mm$^3$), which is analogous to the measurement of mucus cellularity (Section 5.3.5).

Sperm motility in cervical mucus is graded as follows: a, = rapid progressive motility; b, = slow or sluggish progressive motility; c, = non-progressive motility; and d, = immotile spermatozoa (Section 2.4.3). The most important indicator of normal cervical function is the presence of any spermatozoa with rapid progressive motility.

(vi) *Interpretation*  The purpose of a postcoital test is not only to determine the number of active spermatozoa in the cervical mucus but also to evaluate sperm survival and behaviour many hours after coitus (reservoir role). Therefore, a test performed 9–24 hours postcoitally provides information on the longevity and survival of spermatozoa.

The presence of any spermatozoa with rapid progressive motility at this stage in the endocervix argues against significant cervical factors as possible causes of infertility (Oei et al., 1995).

The postcoital test should be repeated if the initial result is negative or abnormal. When no spermatozoa are found in the cervical canal or vagina, the couple should be asked to confirm that ejaculation and deposition of spermatozoa into the vagina have occurred. A negative test may also be due to incorrect timing. A test performed too early or too late in the menstrual cycle may be negative in an otherwise fertile woman. In some women the test may be positive for only 1 or 2 days during the entire menstrual cycle. When ovulation cannot be timed with a reasonable degree of accuracy, it may be necessary to repeat the postcoital test several times during a cycle or to perform repeated tests in vitro. Repeated abnormal postcoital tests in cycles with optimal timing are required to establish cervical factors as a possible cause of infertility.

### 5.4.2 *In vitro tests*

A detailed assessment of sperm–cervical mucus interaction may be undertaken using in vitro penetration tests. These tests are usually performed after there is an abnormal postcoital test, and are most informative when carried out with crossover testing using donor semen and donor cervical mucus.

When the purpose of the sperm–cervical mucus interaction test is to compare the quality of various cervical mucus specimens, a single sample of semen with optimum count, motility, and morphology should be used. On the other hand, when the interest is to evaluate the quality of several semen specimens, the same sample of cervical mucus should be used to assess the ability of spermatozoa to penetrate it. When an abnormal result is obtained using the husband's semen and the wife's mucus, crossover testing using donor semen and donor cervical mucus can be performed to identify whether the semen and/or cervical mucus is responsible for the abnormal result. Donor cervical mucus can be obtained at mid-cycle from women who are scheduled for artificial insemination. The cervical mucus should be collected prior to insemination in natural cycles or cycles in which ovulation is induced by treatment with gonadotrophins. Women who are receiving clomiphene citrate for induction of ovulation should not be used as cervical mucus donors because of the possible effects of this antioestrogen on the cervix.

In vitro tests should be done within 1 hour of semen collection and mid-cycle human cervical mucus should be used. Surrogate gels such as bovine cervical mucus or synthetic gels cannot be regarded as equivalent to human cervical mucus for in vitro testing of sperm–cervical mucus interaction.

(i) *Simplified slide test*  A drop of cervical mucus is placed on a slide and flattened by a cover slip (22 mm × 22 mm). The depth of this preparation can be standardized by supporting the cover slip with silicone grease containing 100 μm glass beads (Section 5.3.5). A drop of semen is deposited at each side and in contact with the edge of the cover slip so that the semen moves under the cover slip by capillary force. In this way a clear interface is obtained between the cervical mucus and the semen.

The slide preparation is incubated at 37 °C in a moist chamber for 30 minutes.

At the interface, finger-like projections (phalanges) of seminal fluid develop within a few minutes and penetrate into the mucus. Most spermatozoa penetrate the phalangeal canal before entering the mucus. In many instances, a single spermatozoon appears to lead a column of sperm into the mucus. Once in the cervical mucus, the spermatozoa fan out and move at random. Some return to the seminal plasma, while most migrate deep into the cervical mucus until they meet resistance from cellular debris or leukocytes.

(ii) *Interpretation*  Interpretation of the simplified slide test is subjective, because it is impossible to standardize the size and shape of the semen–mucus interface in a plain slide preparation. Consequently, it is recommended that the test be used only as a qualitative assessment of sperm–mucus interaction.

Useful observations from the test are as follows:

(a)  Spermatozoa penetrate into the mucus phase and more than 90% are motile with definite progression (normal result).

(b)  Spermatozoa penetrate into the mucus phase, but most do not progress further than 500 μm (i.e., about 10 sperm lengths) from the semen–mucus interface (poor result).

(c)  Spermatozoa penetrate into the mucus phase but rapidly become either immotile or show the 'shaking' pattern of movement (abnormal result, suggesting the presence of antispermatozoal antibodies).

(d)  No penetration of spermatozoa through the semen–mucus interface takes place. Phalanges may or may not be formed, but the spermatozoa congregate along the semen side of the interface (abnormal result).

(iii) *The capillary tube test*  (see Appendix XXI)

# Reference values of semen variables

Each laboratory should determine its own reference range for each variable. For reference semen variables, specimens should be evaluated from men who have recently achieved a pregnancy, preferably within 12 months of the couple ceasing contraception, or prospective studies of fertility should be undertaken. The need for large numbers (around 1000) and the complex relationship between semen analysis results and fertilization, together with the time taken to achieve pregnancy, make these studies difficult to perform. Thus, true reference ranges have not been established as they have for other laboratory tests. To date, no significant differences in semen variables have been found between races.

It should be emphasized again that this manual is not only intended for laboratories dealing with infertility but also addresses the needs of laboratories investigating potential methods for male fertility regulation or studying male reproductive toxicology. In this context the following reference ranges are given, based on the clinical experience of many investigators who have studied populations of healthy fertile men. Because these values are not the minimum semen values needed for conception, e.g., obtained by evaluation of in vitro or in vivo fertility in a subfertile population, their categorization has been changed from 'normal' values to 'reference' values. Thus men with semen variables lower than those indicated in this manual may be fertile.

The following reference values give the description of a semen sample analysed according to the methods described in this manual.

## Reference values

| | |
|---|---|
| Volume | 2.0 ml or more |
| pH | 7.2 or more |
| Sperm concentration | $20 \times 10^6$ spermatozoa/ml or more |
| Total sperm number | $40 \times 10^6$ spermatozoa per ejaculate or more |
| Motility | 50% or more motile (grades a + b) or 25% or more with progressive motility (grade a) within 60 minutes of ejaculation |
| Morphology | * |
| Vitality | 50% or more live, i.e., excluding dye |

| White blood cells | Fewer than $1 \times 10^6$/ml |
| Immunobead test | Fewer than 50% motile spermatozoa with beads bound |
| MAR test | Fewer than 50% motile spermatozoa with adherent particles |

\* Multicentre population-based studies utilizing the methods of morphology assessment in this manual are now in progress.

Data from assisted reproductive technology programmes suggest that, as sperm morphology falls below 15% normal forms using the methods and definitions described in this manual, the fertilization rate in vitro decreases.

# Nomenclature for some semen variables

Since it is often useful to describe deviations from reference semen variables with words instead of numbers, a nomenclature was introduced (Eliasson et al., 1970). It is important to recognize that this nomenclature describes only some semen variables and does not imply any causal relationship. With this stipulation, the nomenclature should be used as follows:

| | |
|---|---|
| Normozoospermia | Normal ejaculate as defined by the reference values |
| Oligozoospermia | Sperm concentration less than the reference value |
| Asthenozoospermia | Less than the reference value for motility |
| Teratozoospermia | Less than the reference value for morphology |
| Oligoasthenoterato-<br>zoospermia | Signifies disturbance of all three variables<br>(combinations of only two prefixes may also be used) |
| Azoospermia | No spermatozoa in the ejaculate |
| Aspermia | No ejaculate |

## Reference

Eliasson, R., Hellinga, F., Lubcke, F., Meyhofer, W., Niermann, H., Steeno, O. & Schirren, C. (1970) Empfehlungen zur Nomenklatur in der Andrologie. *Andrologia,* 2: 1257.

# Safety guidelines for the andrology laboratory[a]

### Conduct of laboratory personnel

1. Human fluids such as semen and blood must be regarded as potentially infectious and should therefore be handled and disposed of with special care.

2. Semen samples could be contaminated with infectious microorganisms or pathogens, and for the andrology laboratory, the most important are the Human Immunodeficiency Virus (HIV) and the Hepatitis B virus (HBV).

3. All personnel working in the andrology laboratory should be vaccinated against hepatitis B.

4. Strict precautions must be taken to avoid accidental wounds from sharp instruments contaminated with semen and the contact of semen with open skin, cuts, abrasions, or lesions.

5. All sharp objects (needles, blades, etc.) should be placed in a marked container, which is sealed before being too full and disposed of in the same way as other dangerous laboratory items. Other disposable items (gloves, semen containers) should be collected for disposal.

6. Infection in the andrology laboratory could also occur following spillage or splashing of infected semen or blood samples. Steps should be taken to prevent and contain spillages.

7. The last drops of the specimens should not be forcibly expelled because this may create droplets or aerosols. Surgical masks must be worn when procedures are conducted that have a potential for creating aerosols or droplets. These include vortexing and centrifuging of open containers.

8. Disposable rubber or plastic gloves must be worn when handling fresh and frozen semen or seminal plasma and any containers that have come into contact with semen or seminal plasma. Gloves must be removed and discarded when leaving the laboratory or when handling the telephone and door handles. Gloves must not be reused.

9. A laboratory coat or disposable gown must be worn in the andrology laboratory. This coat or gown must be removed on leaving the andrology laboratory. Such clothing should not be worn outside the laboratory, especially in social rooms or cafeterias.

[a] Adapted from: Schrader, S.M. (1989) Safety guidelines for the andrology laboratory. *Fertility and Sterility*, **51**: 387–9.

10. Disinfectant soap or antiseptic skin cleanser should be readily available in the laboratory, and personnel should wash their hands regularly, especially before leaving the laboratory, after handling specimens and after removing gowns and gloves.

11. If the outside of a semen collection jar is contaminated, it must be washed with a disinfectant solution (e.g., 5.25 g/l sodium hypochlorite, or household bleach diluted 1:10).

12. Laboratory work surfaces, which should be impermeable, must be decontaminated with a disinfectant (e.g., 5.25g/l sodium hypochlorite, or household bleach diluted 1:10) immediately after any spills occur and also on completing the analyses each day.

13. Disposable laboratory supplies should be used whenever possible and carefully disposed of.

14. Mechanical pipetting devices must be used for the manipulation of liquids in the laboratory. Pipetting by mouth is never permitted.

15. An andrology laboratory should carry equipment for rinsing the eyes.

16. Reagents, chemicals, or dyes of a toxic nature should be kept in a fume cupboard.

17. Eating, drinking, smoking, applying cosmetics, storing food, etc., must not be permitted in the andrology laboratory.

For further details, the reader is referred to two WHO publications: *Laboratory Biosafety Manual*, Geneva, World Health Organization, 1983; and *Guidelines on Sterilization and High-level Disinfection Methods Effective Against Human Immunodeficiency Virus*, 2nd ed., Geneva, World Health Organization, 1989 (AIDS Series, No. 2) p. 10.

# Methods for detecting leukocytes

The traditional method for counting leukocytes in human semen is to use a histochemical procedure to identify the peroxidase enzyme that characterizes polymorphonuclear granulocytes (Fig. 2.4($a$)). This technique has the advantage of being relatively easy to perform, but it does not detect activated polymorphs that have released their granules; nor does it detect other species of leukocyte, such as lymphocytes, that do not contain peroxidase. Such cells can be detected by immunocytochemical means.

### III.1 Peroxidase stain using ortho-toluidine[a]

*III.1.1 Reagents*

1. Saturated $NH_4Cl$ solution (250 g/l)
2. $Na_2EDTA$, 50 g/l in phosphate buffer (pH 6.0)
3. *Ortho*-toluidine, (0.25 mg/ml)[b]
4. $H_2O_2$, 30% in distilled water

The working solution consists of: 1 ml of reagent 1; 1 ml of reagent 2; 9 ml of reagent 3; and one drop of reagent 4.

This solution can be used for 24 hours after preparation.

*III.1.2 Procedure*

(i) Mix 0.1 ml semen with 0.9 ml working solution.
(ii) Shake for 2 minutes.
(iii) Leave for 20–30 minutes at room temperature.
(iv) Shake again.
(v) Peroxidase-positive cells are stained brown, while peroxidase-negative cells are unstained.
(vi) Count in duplicate 200 leukocytes in a haemocytometer chamber and estimate the percentage of peroxidase positive and negative cells.

---

[a] From Nahoum, C.R.D. & Cardozo, D. (1980) Staining for volumetric count of leukocytes in semen and prostate-vesicular fluid. *Fertility and Sterility*, **34**:68–9.

[b] The International Agency for Research on Cancer (IARC) has stated that *ortho*-toluidine 'should be regarded, for practical purposes, as if it presented a carcinogenic risk to humans' (*IARC Monographs on the Evaluation of the Carcinogenic Risk of Chemicals to Humans* (1982), vol. 27, suppl. 4, pp. 169–70).

### III.2  Immunocytochemistry

All classes of human leukocytes express a specific antigen (CD45) that can be detected using an appropriate monoclonal antibody (see Fig. 2.4(b)). By changing the nature of the first antibody, this general procedure can be adapted to allow detection of the different types of leukocyte such as macrophages, neutrophils, B- or T- cells.

*III.2.1  Reagents*

1.  Dulbecco's phosphate buffered saline (PBS).
    Constituents of PBS solution

    | | |
    |---|---|
    | $CaCl_2.2H_2O$ | 0.132 g |
    | KCl | 0.2 g |
    | $KH_2PO_4$ | 0.2 g |
    | $MgCl_2.6H_2O$ | 0.1 g |
    | NaCl | 8.0 g |
    | $Na_2HPO_4$ | 1.15 g |
    | Make up to 1 litre with water. | |

2.  Tris buffered saline (TBS): a $10\times$ stock solution is prepared and diluted 1:10 immediately before use.
    Constituents of $10\times$ TBS solution

    | | |
    |---|---|
    | Trizma base | 60.55 g |
    | NaCl | 85.2 g |
    | Add water, adjust to pH 8.6 with 1 (mol/l) HCl | |
    | Make up to 1 litre with water. | |

3.  Alkaline phosphatase substrate is prepared as described below and filtered.
    Constituents of alkaline phosphatase substrate

    | | |
    |---|---|
    | Naphthol AS-MX phosphate | 2 mg |
    | Dimethylformamide | 0.2 ml |
    | 0.1 M Tris buffer, pH 8.2[a] | 9.7 ml |
    | 1 M Levamisole | 0.1 ml |
    | Fast Red TR salt, added just before use | 10 mg |

    [a]  1.21 g of Trizma base dissolved in water, pH adjusted to 8.2 with 1 M HCl, made up to 100 ml with water.

4.  Primary antibody. A mouse monoclonal antibody against the common leukocyte antigen, encoded CD45, and widely available commercially.
5.  Secondary antibody. Antimouse immunoglobulins raised in a rabbit; the dilution used will depend on antibody titre and source (e.g., 1:25 dilution of the Z259 antibody manufactured by DAKO Corp., 6392 Via Real, Carpinteria, CA 93013, USA).

6. Alkaline phosphatase:antialkaline phosphatase complex (APAAP). Again the dilution will depend on antibody titre and source (e.g., 1:50 dilution of the D651 complex produced by DAKO Corp., 6392 Via Real, Carpinteria, CA 93013, USA).

### III.2.2 Cell preparation
*Procedure*

(i) An aliquot of liquefied semen (approximately 0.5 ml) is mixed with five volumes of phosphate-buffered saline (PBS) and centrifuged at 500*g* for 5 minutes at room temperature.

This procedure is repeated two times and the cell pellet resuspended in PBS to the original volume of the semen sample. The suspension is then diluted with two to five times its volume of PBS depending on the concentration of spermatozoa.

Two 5 μl aliquots of this cell suspension are then air-dried onto a clean glass slide, fixed and stained immediately or wrapped in aluminium foil and stored at $-70\,^{\circ}\mathrm{C}$ until subsequent analysis.

(ii) The air-dried cells are fixed in absolute acetone for 10 minutes or in a mixture of acetone, methanol, and 37% formaldehyde (in volumetric proportions 95:95:10) for 90 seconds, washed twice with Tris buffered saline (TBS; see III.2.1), and allowed to drain.

(iii) Each aliquot of fixed cells is covered with 10 μl of primary monoclonal antibody and incubated in a humidified chamber for 30 minutes at room temperature. The slides are then washed a further 2 × with TBS and allowed to drain.

(iv) The cells are covered with 10 μl of secondary antibody, incubated for 30 minutes in a humidified chamber at room temperature, washed 2 × with TBS and drained.

(v) To each specimen is added 10 μl alkaline phosphatase:anti-alkaline phosphatase complex (APAAP), and the specimen is incubated for 1 hour in a humidified chamber at room temperature before being washed 2 × in TBS and drained.

(vi) In order to intensify the reaction product, staining with the secondary antibody and APAAP can be repeated, with a 15-minute incubation period for each reagent.

(vii) The cells are washed 2 × with TBS, drained, and incubated with 10 μl of alkaline phosphatase substrate for 18 minutes.

(viii) After the alkaline phosphatase colour reaction has developed, the slides are washed with TBS and finally counterstained for a few seconds with haematoxylin before being washed in tap water and mounted in an aqueous mounting medium.

# Sperm vitality techniques

These tests provide a good internal control of the estimate of motility. The sum of dead and motile spermatozoa should not exceed 100%.

## IV.1 Eosin alone

### IV.1.1 Reagents
Eosin Y; make a 5 g/l solution of Eosin Y (Colour Index, C.I. 45380) in a 9 g/L aqueous sodium chloride solution. Alternatively, the standard stain can be obtained from a number of companies in different countries.

### IV.1.2 Procedure
(i) *Either*: Mix one drop of fresh semen with one drop of the eosin solution on a microscope slide, cover with a cover slip and examine after 30 seconds at 400× with a light microscope.

These slides have to be assessed immediately: live spermatozoa are unstained (white); dead cells are stained red.

*Or*: Mix the semen and eosin on a microscope slide and after 1 minute make a smear and air dry. This can be examined later under oil immersion (1000 ×) with a negative phase contrast microscope.

Live spermatozoa appear black and the dead spermatozoa are stained yellow.

(ii) Count unstained (live) and stained (dead) spermatozoa as described in the text (Section 2.5.1).

## IV.2 Eosin–nigrosin (a modification of Blom's technique)

### IV.2.1 Reagents
(i) Eosin Y (C.I. 45380), 10 g/l, in distilled water, i.e., 1%
(ii) Nigrosin (C.I. 50420), 100 g/l, in distilled water, i.e., 10%

### IV.2.2 Procedure
(i) Mix one drop of semen with two drops of 1% Eosin Y.
(ii) After 30 seconds, add three drops of 10% nigrosin solution and mix.
(iii) Place a drop of the semen–eosin–nigrosin mixture on a microscope slide and make a smear within 30 seconds of adding the nigrosin. The

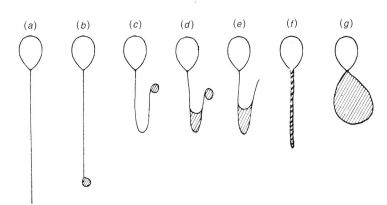

Fig. IV.1. Schematic representation of typical morphological changes of human spermatozoa subjected to hypo-osomotic stress: (a) = no change: (b–g) = various types of tail changes. Tail region showing swelling is indicated by the hatched area.

smears should not be too thick. Allow to air-dry and examine under oil immersion (1000×) with a light microscope.

The live spermatozoa are white and the dead are stained red. The nigrosin provides a dark background which makes the slides easier to assess.

### IV.3    Hypo-osmotic swelling (HOS) test

#### IV.3.1    Swelling solution
Dissolve 0.735 g sodium citrate dihydrate $Na_3C_6H_5O_7.2H_2O$ and 1.351 g fructose in 100 ml distilled water. Store aliquots of this solution frozen at $-20\,^{\circ}C$. Thaw and mix well before use.

#### IV.3.2    Method
Warm 1 ml swelling solution in a closed Eppendorf tube at $37\,^{\circ}C$ for about 5 minutes. Add 0.1 ml liquefied semen and mix gently with the pipette. Keep at $37\,^{\circ}C$ for at least 30 minutes (but not longer than 120 minutes) and examine the sperm cells with a phase-contrast microscope. Swelling of sperm is identified as changes in the shape of the tail, as shown in Fig. IV.1. Count in duplicate the number of swollen cells in a total of 200 spermatozoa counted and calculate the mean percentage.

#### IV.3.3    Interpretation of results
The HOS test is considered normal for a semen sample if more than 60% of the spermatozoa undergo tail swelling. If less than 50% of the spermatozoa show tail swelling, the semen specimen is considered to be abnormal.

Since some semen samples will have spermatozoa with curled tails before exposure to the HOS solution, it is essential that an ejaculate be observed before exposure to the HOS solution. The percentage of spermatozoa with curled tails in the untreated sample should be sub-

tracted from the percentage obtained after treatment to obtain the
true percentage of spermatozoa that reacted in the HOS test.

IV.3.4 *Quality control*

New batches of HOS solution should be checked against the old batch
and scores should not be significantly different ($p>0.05$ by paired
t-test) before being accepted for clinical use. If the difference
is significant, discard the new batch and prepare another solution.

**References**

Eliasson, R. & Treschl, L. (1971) Supravital staining of human spermatozoa. *Fertility and Sterility*, **22**:134–7.

Eliasson, R. (1981) Analysis of semen. In *The Testis*, ed. H. Burger &
D. de Kretser, pp. 381–99. New York: Raven Press.

Jeyendran, R.S., Van der Ven, H.H., Perez-Pelaez, M., Crabo, B.G. &
Zaneveld, L.J.D. (1984) Development of an assay to assess the functional integrity of the human sperm membrane and its relationship
to other semen characteristics. *Journal of Reproduction and Fertility*,
**70**: 219–28.

# Papanicolaou staining procedure modified for spermatozoa

The Papanicolaou stain distinguishes clearly between basophilic and acidophilic cell components and allows a detailed examination of the nuclear chromatin pattern. Although this method has been used for routine diagnostic cytology, the standard Papanicolaou method for vaginal cytology gives poor results when applied to spermatozoa. The present modified staining technique has proved useful in the analysis of sperm morphology and in the examination of immature germ cells (see Figs. 2.9 and 2.11).

### V.1 Preparation of specimen

The smear (see Section 2.5.3) should be air-dried and then fixed in equal parts of 95% (950 ml/l) ethanol and ether for 5–15 minutes.

### V.2 Staining procedure

Fixed smears should be stained by the following procedure:

| | |
|---|---|
| ethanol 80%[a] | 10 dips[b] |
| ethanol 70% | 10 dips |
| ethanol 50% | 10 dips |
| distilled water (deionized, demineralized) | 10 dips |
| Harris's or Mayer's haematoxylin | 3 minutes exactly |
| running water | 3–5 minutes |
| acid ethanol | 2 dips |
| running water | 3–5 minutes |
| Scott's solution[c] | 4 minutes |
| distilled water | 1 dip |
| ethanol 50% | 10 dips |
| ethanol 70% | 10 dips |
| ethanol 80% | 10 dips |
| ethanol 90% | 10 dips |
| Orange G6[d] | 2 minutes |
| ethanol 95% | 10 dips |
| ethanol 95% | 10 dips |
| EA-50[d] | 5 minutes |
| ethanol 95% | 5 dips |
| ethanol 95% | 5 dips |
| ethanol 95% | 5 dips |
| ethanol 99.5% | 2 minutes |
| Xylene[e] or Rotisol[f] (three staining jars) | 1 minute in each |

<sup>a</sup> Check the acidity of the water before preparing the different grades of ethanol. The pH should be 7.0.

<sup>b</sup> One dip corresponds to an immersion of about 1 second.

<sup>c</sup> Scott's solution (see Section V.3.4) is used when the ordinary tap water is 'hard'.

<sup>d</sup> Stains and solutions: the prepared Papanicolaou stain (EA-50 and Orange G6) may be obtained commercially. The same companies usually manufacture the haematoxylin preparation.

<sup>e</sup> Change the xylene if it turns milky. Mount at once with DPX (BDH 36029) or any mounting medium (e.g., Eukitt, Riedel de Haen, D-30926, Germany ). Xylene is not permitted in some countries because of the health risk on inhalation.

<sup>f</sup> Carl Roth GmbH & Co, Schoemperstrasse 1–5, D-76185, Karlsruhe, Germany.

### V.3    Preparation of stains

The commercially available stains are usually satisfactory, but the stains may be prepared in the laboratory at a substantial saving as follows:

### V.3.1    Constituents of EA-36 equivalent to EA-50

| | |
|---|---|
| Eosin Y (Colour Index, C.I. 45380) | 10 g |
| Bismarck Brown Y (C.I. 21000) | 10 g |
| Light-Green SF, Yellowish (C.I. 42095) | 10 g |
| Distilled water | 300 ml |
| Ethanol 95% | 2000 ml |
| Phosphotungstic acid | 4 g |
| Saturated lithium carbonate solution (in distilled water) | 0.5 ml |

### V.3.1.1    Procedure

*Stock solutions*

(i)    Prepare separate 10% solutions of each of the stains as follows:
10 g of Eosin Y in 100 ml of distilled water.
10 g of Bismarck Brown Y in 100 ml of distilled water.
10 g of Light-Green SF in 100 ml of distilled water.

(ii)    To prepare 2 litres of stain, mix the above stock solutions as follows:
50 ml of Eosin Y
10 ml of Bismarck Brown Y
12.5 ml of Light-Green SF

(iii)    Make up to 2 litres with 95% ethanol; add 4 g of phosphotungstic acid and 0.5 ml of saturated lithium carbonate solution.

(iv)    Mix well and store solution at room temperature in dark-brown tightly capped bottles. The solution is stable for 2 to 3 months. Filter before using.

### V.3.2    Constituents of Orange G6

| | |
|---|---|
| Orange G crystals (C.I.16230) | 10 g |
| Distilled water | 100 ml |
| 95% ethanol | 1000 ml |
| Phosphotungstic acid | 0.15 g |

*Procedure*

*Stock solution No. 1 (Orange G6, 10% solution)*

Prepare 10% aqueous solution by dissolving 10 g of Orange G crystals in 100 ml of distilled water. Shake well and allow to stand in a dark-brown bottle at room temperature for 1 week before using.

*Stock solution No. 2 (Orange G6, 0.5% solution)*

Prepare as follows:

(i)    Stock solution No. 1, 50 ml.

(ii)   Make up with 95% ethanol to 1000 ml.

(iii)  Add 0.15 g of phosphotungstic acid.

(iv)  Mix well and store in dark-brown stoppered bottles at room temperature. Filter before use. The solution is stable for 2 to 3 months.

*V.3.3    Constituents of Harris's haematoxylin without acetic acid*

| | |
|---|---|
| Haematoxylin (dark crystals; C.I. 75290) | 8 g |
| 95% ethanol | 80 ml |
| $AlNH_4(SO_4)_2.12H_2O$ | 160 g |
| Distilled water | 1600 ml |
| HgO | 6 g |

*V.3.4    Procedure for preparation of the staining mixture*

(i)    Dissolve 160 g aluminium ammonium sulfate in 1600 ml distilled water by heating.

(ii)   Dissolve 8 g haematoxylin crystals in 80 ml 95% ethanol.

(iii)  Add haematoxylin solution to the aluminium ammonium sulfate solution.

(iv)  Heat the mixture to 95 °C.

(v)   Remove mixture from heat and slowly add the mercuric oxide while stirring. Solution will be dark purple in colour.

(vi)  Immediately plunge the container into a cold water bath and filter when the solution is cold.

(vii) Store in dark-brown bottles at room temperature and allow to stand for 48 hours.

(viii) Dilute the required amount with an equal part of distilled water and filter again.

*V.3.5    Constituents of Scott's solution*

| | |
|---|---|
| $NaHCO_3$ | 3.5 g |
| $MgSO_4.7H_2O$ | 20.0 g |
| Distilled water | 1000 ml |

Scott's solution is to be used only when the ordinary tap water is 'hard' and should be changed frequently, e.g., after rinsing 20 to 25 slides.

## V.3.6 Constituents of acid ethanol solution

| | |
|---|---|
| Ethanol 99.5% | 300 ml |
| Concentrated HCl | 2.0 ml |
| Distilled water | 100 ml |

# Shorr staining procedure for sperm morphology

See Fig. 2.10

### VI.1 Preparation of smear

The smear (see Section 2.5.3) should be air-dried and then fixed in 75% ethanol for about 1 minute.

### VI.2 Staining procedure

Smears should be stained by the following procedure:

| | |
|---|---|
| running water | 12–15 dips[a] |
| haematoxylin | 1–2 minutes |
| running water | 12–15 dips |
| ammonium alcohol | 5 passages of 5 seconds each |
| running water | 12–15 dips |
| 50% ethanol | 5 minutes |
| Shorr stain | 3–5 minutes |
| 50% ethanol | 5 minutes |
| 75% ethanol | 5 minutes |
| 95% ethanol | 5 minutes |
| absolute ethanol | 2 passages of 5 minutes each |
| xylene | 2 passages of 5 minutes each |

[a] One dip corresponds to an immersion of about 1 second.

### VI.3 Reagents

1. Haematoxylin Papanicolaou No. 1 (Merck, Cat. No. 9253).
2. Ammonium alcohol
   95 ml 75% ethanol + 5 ml 25% ammonium hydroxide
3. Either (i) Shorr solution (Merck, Cat. No. 9275)
   or (ii) 4 g BDH Shorr powder (BDH 34147-26) dissolved in 220 ml of warm 50% ethanol and allowed to cool, with addition of 2.0 ml glacial acetic acid (in fume cupboard) and subsequent filtration.

| Concentration ($10^6$/ml) | Motility (grades a + b)%[a] | Semen required[b] (ml) |
|---|---|---|
| >50 | | 0.2 |
| 20–50 | >40 | 0.4 |
| 20–50 | <40 | 0.8 |
| <20 | >40 | 1.0 |
| <20 | <40 | 2.0 |
| <10 | | >2.0 |

[a] See Section 2.4.3.
[b] Aliquots of >1.0 ml require 3 washes.

(iii) Centrifuge all the tubes at $500g$ for 5–10 minutes.

(iv) Sperm tube(s): decant and discard the supernatant. Gently resuspend the sperm pellet in 10 ml of fresh Buffer I and centrifuge again at $500g$ for 5–10 minutes. Decant and discard the supernatant. Gently resuspend the sperm pellet in 0.2 ml of Buffer II.

(v) Immunobead tube(s): decant and discard the supernatant. Gently resuspend the beads in 0.2 ml of Buffer II.

(vi) Place 5 µl drops of each type of immunobead on one or more glass slides. Add 5 µl of the washed sperm suspension to each of the bead drops and mix well using either a pipette tip or the edge of a cover slip. Place a cover slip (20 to 24 mm square) on each of the mixtures, and after leaving the slide for 10 minutes in a moist chamber, observe at $400\times$ to $500\times$ magnification with a phase-contrast microscope.

(vii) Score separately the percentage of *motile* spermatozoa that have two or more attached immunobeads (ignore tail-tip binding). Count at least 200 motile spermatozoa in duplicate per preparation. Record the class (IgG or IgA) and the site of binding of the immunobeads to the spermatozoa (head, mid-piece, tail).

*Interpretation.* The test is regarded as clinically significant if 50% or more of motile (progressive and nonprogressive) spermatozoa are coated with beads. Binding to the tail-tip is not considered to be clinically relevant.

## VIII.3 Indirect immunobead test

The indirect immunobead test is used to detect antisperm antibodies in heat inactivated serum, seminal plasma, or bromelain-solubilized cervical mucus.

(i) Wash normal donor spermatozoa twice with Buffer I as described above, steps (ii), (iii), (iv).

(ii) Adjust the washed sperm suspension to a concentration of $50 \times 10^6$/ml in Buffer II.

(iii) Dilute 10 µl of the body fluid to be tested with 40 µl of Buffer II and then mix with 50 µl of the washed sperm suspension. Incubate at 37 °C for 1 hour.

(iv) Wash the spermatozoa twice again as described above, steps (iii) and (iv), and perform the tests as described in steps (vi) and (vii).

## VIII.4 Controls

A positive control and a negative control should be included in each test run. A positive control can be prepared using serum from a donor (e.g., a vasectomized man) with high titres of serum sperm antibodies as detected by the indirect immunobead test. This serum is prepared as in VIII.3 and assayed in parallel with each test run.

### References

Bronson, R.A., Cooper, G.W. & Rosenfeld, D. (1982) Detection of sperm specific antibodies on the spermatozoa surface by immunobead binding. *Archives of Andrology*, **9**: 61.

Bronson, R.A., Cooper, G.W. & Rosenfeld, D. (1984) Sperm antibodies: their role in infertility. *Fertility and Sterility*, **42**: 171–83.

Clarke, G.N., Stojanoff, A. & Cauchi, M.N. (1982) Immunoglobulin class of sperm-bound antibodies in semen. In *Immunology of Reproduction*, ed. K. Bratanov, pp. 482–5. Sofia, Bulgaria: Bulgarian Academy of Sciences Press.

Clarke, G.N. (1990) Detection of antisperm antibodies using Immunobeads. In *Handbook of the Laboratory Diagnosis and Treatment of Infertility*, ed. B.A. Keel & B.W. Webster, pp. 177–92. Boca Raton, Florida: CRC.

# Mixed antiglobulin reaction test (MAR test)

Since IgA antibodies almost never occur without IgG antibodies, testing for the latter is sufficient as a routine screening method. Reagents for the MAR test are available from Fertility Technologies, Natick, Massachusetts 017601, USA and from Fertipro N.V., Beernem, Belgium.

## IX.1 Procedure

(i) 10 µl of unwashed fresh semen, 10 µl of IgG- and IgA-coated latex particles (from Fertility Technologies Inc.) and 10 µl of antiserum to human IgG (from Hoechst-Behring ORCM-04/05, or Dakopatts A089, Denmark) or human IgA are placed on a microscope slide.

(ii) The drops of semen and IgG (or IgA)-coated particles are mixed first, and then the drop of antiserum is added using a larger cover slip (e.g., 40 mm × 24 mm), which is then laid on the mixture. The wet preparation is observed in the microscope at 400× or 600× magnification either using bright field or phase contrast optics after 2–3 minutes and again after 10 minutes.

## IX.2 Interpretation

In the absence of coating antibodies, the spermatozoa will be seen swimming freely between the particles, which themselves adhere to each other in groups, proving the effectiveness of the preparation.

If sperm antibodies are present on the spermatozoa, the motile spermatozoa will have latex particles adhering to them. The motile spermatozoa are initially seen moving around with a few or even a bunch of particles attached. Eventually the agglutinates become so massive that the movements of the spermatozoa are severely restricted.

At least 200 motile spermatozoa should be counted. The percentage of the motile spermatozoa that have particles attached is calculated.

# Measurement of zinc in seminal plasma

### X.1 Background

A colorimetric assay for the determination of zinc in body fluids was shown to be useful for the determination of zinc in seminal plasma. The method given is modified from that of Johnson & Eliasson (1987).

A kit for the estimation of zinc in semen is available (from Wako Chemicals GmbH, Nissanstrasse 2, 41468 Neuss 1, Germany). The assay described is for users of a plate reader with 96 wells. The volumes of semen and reagents can be proportionally adjusted for spectrophotometers using 3-ml or 1-ml cuvettes. The appropriate corrections must be made for the calculation of results.

### X.2 Principle

$$5\text{-Br-PAPS} + Zn^{2+} \longrightarrow 5\text{-Br-PAPS-Zn complex, which absorbs at}$$
wavelength 560 nm.

5-Br-PAPS is an abbreviation for 2-(5-bromo-2-pyridylazo)-5-($N$-propyl-$N$-sulphopropylamino)-phenol.

### X.3 Reagents

1. Zinc kit (from Wako Chemicals), which is stable at room temperature for a year. Use only colour reagent A ($2 \times 60$ ml bottles) and colour reagent B ($1 \times 30$ ml bottle).

2. Zinc standard: dissolve 0.144 g $ZnSO_4.7H_2O$ in 50 ml water and dilute this $100\times$ by adding 1 ml to 99 ml water to achieve a concentration of 0.1 mM (0.1 mmol/l); store at room temperature or $-20\,°C$.

### X.4 Method

1. Prepare a standard curve: dilute 100 μM zinc standard with water to yield additional standards of 80, 60, 40, 20 and 10 μM.

2. Prepare colour reagent: mix 4 parts colour reagent A with 1 part colour reagent B (about 25 ml is needed for one 96-well plate). This chromogen solution is stable for 2 days at room temperature or 1 week at 4 °C

3. Sample preparation:

(i) Centrifuge the semen sample for 10 minutes at 1000$g$, decant the seminal plasma and store until analysis at $-20\,°C$.

(ii) Thaw the sperm-free seminal plasma and mix well on a vortex mixer.

(Internal quality control samples containing high, medium, and low concentrations of zinc are also assayed.)

(iii) Dilute each sample of seminal plasma in duplicate: to 300 μl water in a 1.5 ml tube add 5 μl seminal plasma (with a positive displacement pipette) and mix.

(iv) To the 96-well plate add duplicate 40 μl diluted semen samples. Include duplicate blanks (40 μl water) and standards.

(v) Add 200 μl colour reagent and mix for 5 minutes on 96-well-plate shaker.

(vi) Read plate at 560 nm wavelength.

### X.5 Calculation

1. Read the concentration of zinc in the sample from the standard curve (mM).
2. Multiply by the dilution factor (61) to obtain the concentration of zinc (mM) in undiluted seminal plasma.
3. Multiply by ejaculate volume to obtain μmol/ejaculate.
4. Reject samples that lie above the top standard and reassay these samples at greater dilution.

### X.6 Reference value

2.4 μmol or more per ejaculate.

### Reference

Johnson, Ø. & Eliasson, R. (1987) Evaluation of a commercially available kit for the colorimetric determination of zinc in human seminal plasma. *International Journal of Andrology*, **10**: 435–40.

# Measurement of fructose in seminal plasma

### XI.1 Background

The method given is modified from that of Karvonen & Malm (1955). A kit for the estimation of fructose in semen is available (from FertiPro N.V., Lotenhulle, Belgium). The assay described is for users of a 96-well-plate reader. The volumes of semen and reagents can be proportionally adjusted for spectrophotometers using 3-ml or 1-ml cuvettes. The appropriate corrections must be made for the calculation of results.

### XI.2 Principle

$$\text{Fructose} + \text{indole} \xrightarrow{\text{heat, acid}} \text{complex, which absorbs at wavelength } 470 \text{ nm.}$$

### XI.3 Reagents

1. Deproteinizing agents: 63 $\mu$M ($\mu$mol/l) $ZnSO_4.7H_2O$ (dissolve 1.8 g in 100 ml water) and 0.1 M (mol/l)-NaOH (dissolve 0.4 g in 100 ml water).
2. Colour reagent (indole 2 $\mu$M in benzoate preservative 16 $\mu$M): dissolve 200 mg benzoic acid in 90 ml water by shaking in a water bath at 60 °C; dissolve 25 mg indole in this and make up to 100 ml; filter and store at 4 °C.
3. Fructose standard (2.24 mM): dissolve 40.32 mg fructose in 100 ml water; store at 4 °C or freeze in aliquots.

### XI.4 Method

1. Prepare a standard curve: dilute the 2.24 mM standard with water to yield four additional standards of 1.12, 0.56, 0.28 and 0.14 mM.
2. Sample preparation:
   (i) Centrifuge the semen sample for 10 minutes at 1000$g$, decant the seminal plasma and store at −20 °C until analysis.
   (ii) Thaw the sperm-free seminal plasma and mix well on a vortex mixer. (Internal quality control samples containing high, medium and low concentrations of fructose are also assayed.)
   (iii) Dilute each semen sample in duplicate: to 50 $\mu$l water in a 1.5 ml tube add 5 $\mu$l seminal plasma (with a positive displacement pipette) and mix.

(iv) Deproteinize each semen sample: to the 55 μl diluted sample add 12.5 μl 63 μM $ZnSO_4$ and 12.5 μl 0.1M-NaOH, mix, allow to stand for 15 minutes at room temperature and then centrifuge samples at 8000$g$ for 5 minutes.

(v) Remove 50 μl supernatant to test tubes. Include duplicate blanks (50 μl water) and duplicate 50 μl standards.

(vi) Add 50 μl indole reagent to each tube, mix; add 0.5 ml concentrated (32%) HCl to each sample, cover with Parafilm, mix carefully in fume cupboard/hood; heat for 20 minutes at 50 °C in water bath, mix; cool in ice-water (15 minutes)[a].

(vii) Transfer 250 μl with a positive displacement pipette to 96-well plates carefully in fume cupboard/hood.

(viii) Read the plate (with the lid on to protect the spectrophotometer) in a 96-well plate reader at 470 nm wavelength.

## XI.5  Calculation

1. Read the concentration of fructose in the sample from the standard curve (mM).

2. Multiply by the dilution factor (16) to obtain the concentration of fructose (mM) in undiluted seminal plasma.

3. Multiply by the ejaculate volume to obtain μmol/ejaculate.

4. Reject samples that lie above the top standard and reassay these samples at greater dilution.

## XI.6  Reference value

13 μmol or more per ejaculate.

### Reference

Karvonen, M.J. & Malm, M. (1955) Colorimetric determination of fructose with indol. *Scandinavian Journal of Clinical Laboratory Investigation*, 7: 305–7.

---

[a] If the use of concentrated HCl is considered unpleasant, an alternative but more expensive enzymatic assay using ultraviolet spectrophotometry (e.g., Boehringer Mannheim kit No. 139106) may be performed.

# Measurement of neutral $\alpha$-glucosidase in seminal plasma

### XII.1 Background

Seminal plasma contains both a neutral α-glucosidase isoenzyme that originates from the epididymis and an acid isoenzyme contributed by the prostate. The latter can be selectively inhibited (Paquin et al, 1984) to permit measurement of the neutral α-glucosidase reflecting epididymal function. Kits for the estimation of glucosidase in semen are available (from Boehringer Mannheim, Cat. No. 1 742 027, and from FertiPro N.V., Beernem, Belgium). The method given is from Cooper et al. (1990). The assay described is for users of a 96-well-plate reader. The volumes of semen and reagents can be proportionally adjusted for spectrophotometers using 3-ml or 1-ml cuvettes. The appropriate corrections must be made for the calculation of results.

### XII.2 Principle

$$p\text{-nitrophenol-}\alpha\text{-glucopyranoside} \xrightarrow{\quad\alpha\text{-glucosidase}\quad} p\text{-nitrophenol} \xrightarrow{\quad Na_2CO_3\quad}$$

absorbs at 405 nm

### XII.3 Reagents

1. 0.2M (mol/l) phosphate buffer, pH 6.8: prepare from 0.2M- $K_2HPO_4.3H_2O$ (dissolve 4.56 g in 100 ml) and 0.2M- $KH_2PO_4$ (dissolve 2.72 g in 100 ml) and mix approximately equal volumes of each until the pH is 6.8.

2. Buffer containing 1% sodium dodecyl sulphate (SDS): dissolve 1 g SDS in 100 ml of the above buffer. This precipitates on storage at 4 °C, but redissolves upon gentle warming.

3. Colour reagent 1 (for stopping the reaction): 0.1M $Na_2CO_3.H_2O$. Dissolve 6.20 g $Na_2CO_3.H_2O$ in 500 ml water.

4. Colour reagent 2 (for diluting the product): colour reagent 1 containing 0.1% (w/v) SDS.

5. Substrate $p$-nitrophenol glucopyranoside (PNPG), 5 g/l: make freshly for each assay by dissolving 0.1 g PNPG (Sigma N1377) in 20 ml buffer containing 1% SDS and warm the solution on a hot plate at about 50 °C with stirring for about 10 minutes. A few crystals may remain undissolved. The solution should be kept at 37 °C during use.

6. Glucosidase inhibitor for semen blanks (castanospermine): prepare a

10 mM stock by dissolving 0.0189 g castanospermine (Sigma C3784) in 10 ml water and dilute further in water to give a 1 mM working solution. Freeze in aliquots at $-20\,^{\circ}$C.

7. Standard, 5 mM $p$-nitrophenol (PNP): dissolve 0.0695 g PNP (Sigma 104-8) in 100 ml water. Warm the solution if necessary and store at $4\,^{\circ}$C in a brown bottle. Make up a fresh standard solution every three months.

## XII.4 Method

1. Prepare a standard curve (within the last hour of incubation):
   (i) place 400 $\mu$l 5 mM stock PNP in a 10-ml volumetric flask and make up to 10 ml with colour reagent 2 (200 $\mu$M).
   (ii) dilute the 200 $\mu$M standard with colour reagent 2 to yield four additional standards of 160, 120, 80 and 40 $\mu$M PNP.

2. Prepare samples:
   (i) Centrifuge the semen sample for 10 minutes at 1000$g$, decant the seminal plasma and store until analysis at $-20\,^{\circ}$C.
   (ii) Thaw the sperm-free seminal plasma and mix well on a vortex mixer. (Internal quality control samples containing high, medium and low activities of neutral $\alpha$-glucosidase are also assayed.)
   (iii) Place duplicate 15 $\mu$l semen samples with a positive displacement pipette in 1.5 ml tubes. Include duplicate blanks (15 $\mu$l water), duplicate internal quality control semen pools containing medium and low activities of glucosidase and quadruplicate internal quality control semen pools containing high-activity glucosidase.
   (iv) To two of the high-activity quality-control semen pools add 8 $\mu$l of 1 mM castanospermine to provide the semen blank value.
   (v) Place 100 $\mu$l PNPG substrate solution (at about $37\,^{\circ}$C) in each Eppendorf tube.
   (vi) Vortex each tube and incubate at $37\,^{\circ}$C for 2 hours (exact temperature and time control are crucial).
   (vii) Stop incubation after 2 hours by the addition of 1 ml colour reagent 1 and mix.
   (viii) Transfer 250-$\mu$l samples and standards to the 96-well-plate.
   (ix) Read the plate in a 96-well-plate reader at 405 nm wavelength within 60 minutes, using the water blank to set zero.

## XII.5 Calculation

1 unit (U) of glucosidase activity = the production of 1 $\mu$mol product (PNP) per minute at $37\,^{\circ}$C. In this assay the activity is derived from 15 $\mu$l semen in a total volume of 1.115 ml over 120 minutes, so a correction factor of $1115/15/120$ ($=0.6194$) is required.

1. Read the concentration of PNP produced by the sample from the standard curve ($\mu$M).
2. Multiply by the correction factor (0.6194) to obtain the activity of neutral glucosidase in undiluted seminal plasma (U/l).
3. Subtract the activity (U/l) of the castanospermine semen blank from each sample to obtain the corrected (glucosidase-related) activity.
4. Multiply the corrected activity by the ejaculate volume to obtain glucosidase activity (mU) per ejaculate.
5. Reject samples that lie above the top standard and reassay these samples after dilution.

## XII.6 Reference value

20 mU per ejaculate (minimum).

### References

Cooper, T.G., Yeung, C.H., Nashan, D., Jockenhövel, F. & Nieschlag, E. (1990) Improvement in the assessment of human epididymal function by the use of inhibitors in the assay of α-glucosidase in seminal plasma. *International Journal of Andrology,* **13**: 297–305.

Paquin, R., Chapdelaine, P., Dube, J.Y. & Tremblay, R.R. (1984) Similar biochemical properties of human seminal plasma and epididymal α-1,4-glucosidase. *Journal of Andrology,* **5**: 277–82.

# Sample instructions and record form for semen analysis

**A.** **Sample instructions for the collection and delivery of a semen sample**

1. Refrain from sexual intercourse and masturbation for between 2 days and 7 days.

2. Produce the sample by masturbation without artificial lubrication. When collection by masturbation is not possible, special condoms (not ordinary latex condoms; see Section 2.1 (e)) may be used.

3. Collect the sample in a clean, wide-mouth container of glass or plastic. It is important that the whole ejaculate is collected. If not, the sample should be labelled 'incomplete'.

4. Within 1 hour of collection, bring the container and sample to the laboratory, keeping it warm in a pocket near to your body.

5. Samples may also be produced in a room near the laboratory.

6. Label the specimen with name (and/or identification number), date, and time of collection.

**B.** **Sample record form for semen analysis**

This sample record form is offered as a model. It contains a layout for recording the observations made during the semen analysis, using the methods described in this manual. When used for clinical purposes, it may be useful to add certain derived variables, which are combinations of results from the data. An example of such a variable is the total motile sperm count (obtained by multiplying the sperm concentration, the semen volume, and the percentage of motile spermatozoa). Such derived variables have not been included on the sample form since their use depends on the clinical circumstances and the clinician's views of their relevance. When used for research purposes, data from the sample record form can be entered directly into a computer database, and any derived variables can be computed electronically.

The sample record form has been printed with multiple columns for recording the results of semen analyses collected on different dates. This is a convenient way of presenting serial semen sample results. Similarly, additional space may be required in certain places to allow the recording of comments and observations that cannot be coded on the form.

# SAMPLE RECORD FORM FOR SEMEN ANALYSIS

| | Day Month Year | Day Month Year | Day Month Year |
|---|---|---|---|
| Date of sample | ⌊_⌊_⌊_⌊_⌊_⌋ | ⌊_⌊_⌊_⌊_⌊_⌋ | ⌊_⌊_⌊_⌊_⌊_⌋ |
| Duration of abstinence (days) | ⌊_⌊_⌋ | ⌊_⌊_⌋ | ⌊_⌊_⌋ |
| Interval between ejaculation and start of analysis (min) | ⌊_⌊_⌊_⌋ | ⌊_⌊_⌊_⌋ | ⌊_⌊_⌊_⌋ |
| Appearance (1 – normal, 2 – abnormal) | ⌊_⌋ | ⌊_⌋ | ⌊_⌋ |
| Liquefaction (1 – normal, 2 – abnormal) | ⌊_⌋ | ⌊_⌋ | ⌊_⌋ |
| Consistency (1 – normal, 2 – abnormal) | ⌊_⌋ | ⌊_⌋ | ⌊_⌋ |
| Volume (ml) | ⌊_⌊_._⌋ | ⌊_⌊_._⌋ | ⌊_⌊_._⌋ |
| pH | ⌊_._⌋ | ⌊_._⌋ | ⌊_._⌋ |
| Motility (% spermatozoa) | | | |
| (a) rapid progression | ⌊_⌊_⌊_⌋ | ⌊_⌊_⌊_⌋ | ⌊_⌊_⌊_⌋ |
| (b) slow progression | ⌊_⌊_⌊_⌋ | ⌊_⌊_⌊_⌋ | ⌊_⌊_⌊_⌋ |
| (c) non-progressive motility | ⌊_⌊_⌊_⌋ | ⌊_⌊_⌊_⌋ | ⌊_⌊_⌊_⌋ |
| (d) immotile | ⌊_⌊_⌊_⌋ | ⌊_⌊_⌊_⌋ | ⌊_⌊_⌊_⌋ |
| Agglutination (%) | ⌊_⌊_⌊_⌋ | ⌊_⌊_⌊_⌋ | ⌊_⌊_⌊_⌋ |
| Vitality (% live) | ⌊_⌊_⌊_⌋ | ⌊_⌊_⌊_⌋ | ⌊_⌊_⌊_⌋ |
| Concentration ($10^6$/ml) | ⌊_⌊_⌊_⌊_._⌋ | ⌊_⌊_⌊_⌊_._⌋ | ⌊_⌊_⌊_⌊_._⌋ |
| Morphology (%) | | | |
| – normal | ⌊_⌊_⌊_⌋ | ⌊_⌊_⌊_⌋ | ⌊_⌊_⌊_⌋ |
| – head defects | ⌊_⌊_⌊_⌋ | ⌊_⌊_⌊_⌋ | ⌊_⌊_⌊_⌋ |
| – neck or midpiece defects | ⌊_⌊_⌊_⌋ | ⌊_⌊_⌊_⌋ | ⌊_⌊_⌊_⌋ |
| – tail defects | ⌊_⌊_⌊_⌋ | ⌊_⌊_⌊_⌋ | ⌊_⌊_⌊_⌋ |
| – cytoplasmic droplets | ⌊_⌊_⌊_⌋ | ⌊_⌊_⌊_⌋ | ⌊_⌊_⌊_⌋ |
| White blood cells ($10^6$/ml) | ⌊_⌊_._⌋ | ⌊_⌊_._⌋ | ⌊_⌊_._⌋ |
| Immature germ cells ($10^6$/ml) | ⌊_⌊_._⌋ | ⌊_⌊_._⌋ | ⌊_⌊_._⌋ |
| Immunobead/MAR test (% with adherent Ig beads) | ⌊_⌊_⌊_⌋ | ⌊_⌊_⌊_⌋ | ⌊_⌊_⌊_⌋ |
| MAR test (% with adherent particles) | ⌊_⌊_⌊_⌋ | ⌊_⌊_⌊_⌋ | ⌊_⌊_⌊_⌋ |
| Biochemistry | | | |
| zinc (mmol/l) | ⌊_._⌊_⌋ | ⌊_._⌊_⌋ | ⌊_._⌊_⌋ |
| fructose (mmol/l) | ⌊_⌊_._⌋ | ⌊_⌊_._⌋ | ⌊_⌊_._⌋ |
| α-glucosidase (neutral) (U/l) | ⌊_⌊_._⌋ | ⌊_⌊_._⌋ | ⌊_⌊_._⌋ |

# Computer-aided sperm analysis (CASA)

### XIV.1 Systems available

Several commercial manufacturers provide CASA systems, e.g., Hamilton Thorne (Hamilton Thorne Research, Beverly MA, USA), Hobson Sperm Tracker (Hobson Sperm Tracking, Sheffield, United Kingdom) and several versions of each system are available.

### XIV.2 Parameter settings

The correct setup for each CASA instrument is vital for optimum performance and will depend on its anticipated use. The manufacturers provide suitable settings but the user is responsible for checking that each instrument is performing to the required degree of repeatability and reliability. Use of appropriate quality control material, e.g., video-tapes, is essential (see Chapter 4). The following authors have discussed CASA settings in a general context (Davis & Katz, 1992; Mortimer, 1994b).

### XIV.3 Preparation of samples

The criteria for semen collection and preparation for CASA applications are identical to those in Chapter 2. The CASA systems must maintain the specimen temperature at 37 °C because the variables of sperm motion are temperature-sensitive. Motility characteristics and sperm concentration can be assessed in undiluted semen. Often, however, as in samples with high sperm concentrations (i.e., greater than $50 \times 10^6$/ml), collisions may occur with increasing frequency and are likely to induce errors. In such cases, dilution of the sample is recommended. If dilution in homologous seminal plasma is not practical, dilution to a final standard concentration ($25-50 \times 10^6$/ml) with media is acceptable. Dulbecco's PBS-glucose-BSA medium can be used (for discussion of media supporting sperm motility, see Farrell et al., 1996). In order to standardize results, the same dilution medium should be used throughout.

Composition of Dulbecco's PBS-glucose-BSA

|  | (g/l) | (mmol/l) |
|---|---|---|
| NaCl | 8.000 | 137 |
| KCl | 0.200 | 3 |
| CaCl$_2$ (anhydrous)[a] | 0.100 | 1 |
| Na$_2$HPO$_4$ (anhydrous) | 1.150 | 8 |
| KH$_2$PO$_4$ | 0.200 | 1 |
| MgCl$_2$ (anhydrous)[a] | 0.047 | <1 |
| D-Glucose | 1.000 | 6 |
| Phenol red | 0.005 | — |
| Sodium pyruvate | 0.036 | <1 |
| BSA[b] | 3.000 | — |

Also added: 0.4% antibiotic mixture
(GIBCO, Grand Island, New York, USA)

[a] Added separately to prevent precipitation.
[b] BSA Bovine serum albumen (Cat. No. A6003, Sigma Chemical Co., St. Louis, Missouri), essentially fatty acid free, is added last.

Specialized chambers for use in CASA machines are available. A 20 μm-deep Microcell counting chamber (Conception Technologies, San Diego, CA, USA) gives reliable results when analysing spermatozoa in semen. Both chambers should be filled and assessed. Several representative fields should be examined: 6 fields per chamber (12 fields in total) give reliable results. At least 200 spermatozoa in each chamber should be assessed. The same principles of quality control apply as for standard estimations of concentration (see Section 2.5.2). If hyperactivated spermatozoa separated from seminal plasma are to be examined, the depth of chamber should be a minimum of 20 μm.

## XIV.4 Use of the CASA instrument

Samples can either be analysed directly or by means of a video recording. Analysis from a videotape improves standardization and allows implementation of quality assurance procedures (Chapter 4). The manufacturer will advise on the choice of videotape recorder and on the optimum setting of the illumination to achieve maximum contrast between sperm heads and the background.

The time necessary to follow the spermatozoa to achieve accurate results is controversial. The Hamilton Thorne and the Hobson tracker will follow spermatozoa for a minimum of 1 second, which should be sufficient to give reliable determinations of the basic CASA measurements in semen (see Mortimer, 1994b).

## XIV. 5 CASA terminology

There is a standard terminology for variables measured by CASA systems, some of which are illustrated in Fig. XIV.1.

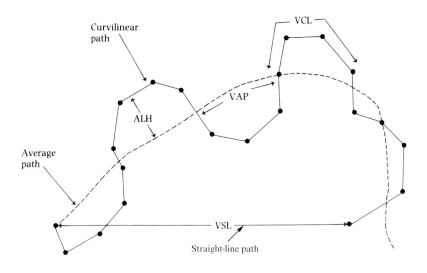

Fig. XIV.1. Standard terminology for variables measured by CASA systems.

VCL = *curvilinear velocity* (μm/s). Time-average velocity of a sperm head along its actual curvilinear path, as perceived in two dimensions in the microscope.

VSL = *straight-line velocity* (μm/s). Time-average velocity of a sperm head along the straight line between its first detected position and its last.

VAP = *average path velocity* (μm/s). Time-average velocity of a sperm head along its average path. This path is computed by smoothing the actual path according to algorithms in the CASA instrument; these algorithms vary between instruments.

ALH = *amplitude of lateral head displacement* (μm). Magnitude of lateral displacement of a sperm head about its average path. It can be expressed as a maximum or an average of such displacements. Different CASA instruments compute ALH using different algorithms, so that values are not strictly comparable.

LIN = *linearity*. The linearity of a curvilinear path, VSL/VCL.

WOB = *wobble*. Measure of oscillation of the actual path about the average path, VAP/VCL.

STR = *straightness*. Linearity of the average path, VSL/VAP.

BCF = *beat-cross frequency* (beats/second). The average rate at which the sperm's curvilinear path crosses its average path.

MAD = *mean angular displacement* (degrees). The time average of absolute values of the instantaneous turning angle of the sperm head along its curvilinear trajectory.

Different CASA instruments use different mathematical algorithms to compute many of these movement variables. The degree of comparability of measurements across all instruments is not yet known.

## XIV. 6 Statistical analysis

It is recommended that computer-aided sperm analysis be used to obtain movement parameters for at least 200 motile sperm tracks per specimen. Note that this will require detection of many more spermatozoa. If it is desired to sort spermatozoa into subcategories of motion or to make other analyses of variability within a specimen, the tracks of at least 200 and, if possible, 400 motile spermatozoa will be needed. Experimental designs should standardize the number of spermatozoa analysed per specimen. It is desirable to interface the CASA instruments with computer software that permits data organization and statistical analysis. The distributions of many of the movement parameters within a specimen are not normal. Therefore the median, rather than the mean value, should be used to summarize the central tendency of each movement variable. It may be necessary to perform mathematical transformations of the measurements for single spermatozoa before certain statistical analyses are done.

### References

(see Bibliography for the references which also appear in Sections 2.11 and 2.14)

Davis, R.O. & Katz, D.F. (1992) Standardization and comparability of CASA instruments. *Journal of Andrology*, **13**: 81–6.

Farrell, P.B., Foote, R.H., McArdle, M.M., Trouern-Trend, V.L. & Tardif, A.L. (1996) Media and dilution procedures tested to minimize handling effects on human, rabbit and bull sperm for computer-assisted sperm analysis (CASA). *Journal of Andrology*, **17**: 293–300.

Mortimer D. (1994b) *Practical Laboratory Andrology.* Oxford: Oxford University Press.

# Protocols for the zona-free hamster oocyte test

## XV.1 Standard protocol

### XV.1.1 Procedure

(i) Allow 30 to 60 minutes for full liquefaction of the semen sample to occur.

(ii) The culture medium for the test is medium BWW (Biggers et al., 1971). This medium is prepared as a stock solution (see below) that can be stored at $4\,°C$ for several weeks without deterioration. On the day of the test, 100 ml of the stock solution is supplemented with 210 mg sodium bicarbonate, 100 mg glucose, 0.37 ml of a 600 g/l sodium lactate syrup, 3 mg sodium pyruvate, 350 mg Fraction V bovine serum albumin, 10 000 units penicillin, 10 mg streptomycin sulfate and 20 mM HEPES salts. The medium should be warmed to $37\,°C$ before use, preferably in an atmosphere of 5% $CO_2$, 95% air.

*Components of the medium BWW stock solution*

| Compound | Quantity g/l |
|---|---|
| NaCl | 5.540 |
| KCl | 0.356 |
| $CaCl_2.2H_2O$ | 0.250 |
| $KH_2PO_4$ | 0.162 |
| $MgSO_4.7H_2O$ | 0.294 |
| Phenol red, 1.0 ml/l | |

(iii) Semen samples are prepared using the sperm preparation techniques described in Appendix XVIII. If the 'swim-up' procedure is used, a number of tubes (three to ten depending on the volume of the sample and the concentration of the spermatozoa in semen) can be prepared.

The tubes are incubated at $37\,°C$ for 1 hour in an atmosphere of 5% $CO_2$, 95% air. If such an incubator is not available, the tubes may be tightly capped and maintained at $37\,°C$ in air. During the incubation period the most motile spermatozoa migrate from the seminal plasma into the overlying medium.

(iv) The sperm suspension is centrifuged at $500g$ for 5 minutes and then resuspended at approximately $10\times10^6$ spermatozoa/ml in a volume of not less than 0.5 ml and incubated for 18–24 hours at 37 °C in an atmosphere of 5% $CO_2$, 95% air. If a $CO_2$ incubator is not available, the tubes can be capped tightly and incubated at 37 °C in air. During the incubation period, the tubes should be inclined at an angle of 20° to the horizontal in order to prevent settling of the spermatozoa into a pellet and to increase the surface area for gaseous exchange.

(v) Oocytes can be obtained from immature hamsters injected at random or from mature hamsters injected on day one of the oestrous cycle. Pregnant mare's serum (PMS) and human chorionic gonadotrophin (hCG) are injected intraperitoneally at a dose of 30 to 40 IU, 48 to 72 hours apart. The oocytes should then be recovered within 18 hours after the injection of hCG and prepared at room temperature using 0.1% hyaluronidase and 0.1% trypsin to remove the cumulus cells and zonae pellucidae, respectively. Each enzyme treatment should be followed by two washes in medium BWW. The isolated oocytes can be warmed to 37 °C and introduced immediately into the sperm suspensions or stored at 4 °C for up to 24 hours.

(vi) At the end of the capacitation phase, the incubation tubes are returned to a vertical position for 20 minutes to allow settling of any immotile cells, after which the motile spermatozoa are aspirated in the supernatant and adjusted to a concentration of $3.5 \times 10^6$ motile spermatozoa/ml. The spermatozoa are then placed under liquid paraffin in 50 to 100 µl droplets, and 30 zona-free hamster oocytes are introduced, incorporating at least 15 oocytes per droplet. The gametes are then incubated at 37 °C in an atmosphere of 5% $CO_2$, 95% air for 3 hours.

(vii) The number of spermatozoa that have entered the oocytes is then assessed by carefully removing the oocytes and washing them free of loosely adherent spermatozoa; after which they are compressed to a depth of about 30 µm beneath a 22 mm × 22 mm cover slip and examined by phase-contrast microscopy. (Fixation and storage of the oocytes in, for example, 1% glutaraldehyde, followed by staining with lacmoid or aceto-orcein, is a possibility.)

(viii) The oocytes should then be examined to determine the percentage that have spermatozoa within their cytoplasm and the mean number of incorporated spermatozoa per oocyte (Fig XV.1). The presence of spermatozoa remaining bound to the surface of the oocyte after the initial washing procedure should also be recorded, since this may give some indication of the proportion of the sperm population that has undergone the acrosome reaction.

### XV.2  Protocol incorporating Ca ionophore (A23187)

A highly motile sperm population is prepared by Percoll gradient centrifugation employing a two-step discontinuous gradient as described in Appendix XVIII. The pellet at the bottom of the 80% fraction is then

Fig. XV.1. A zona-free hamster oocyte containing human spermatozoa, as seen by phase-contrast microsopy. The arrows indicate the presence of decondensing sperm heads within the ooplasm (scale: $\times = 500$). From Aitken et al. (1983).

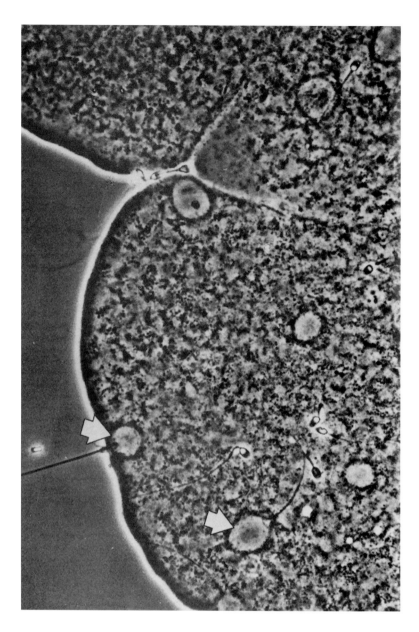

taken up into 8 ml of medium BWW, centrifuged at $500g$ for 5 minutes and finally resuspended at a concentration of $5 \times 10^6$ motile spermatozoa/mL.

A23187 is prepared as follows: a 1 mM suspension of the free acid of A23187 is prepared from a 10 mM stock in dimethylsulfoxide (DMSO) by a 1 in 10 dilution with medium BWW. This suspension is kept at 4 °C for *at least 3 days* before use.

On the day of the test, the A23187 is added to the spermatozoa to achieve two final concentrations of 1.25 and 2.5 μM. The dose–response curve for ionophore treatment varies from individual to individual, and as a result it is preferable to test each patient at both 1.25 and 2.5 $\mu$M. The spermatozoa are incubated with the ionophore for 3 hours, after which the cells are pelleted by centrifugation at $500g$ and resuspended in the same volume of fresh medium BWW.

At this point the percentage of motile spermatozoa is assessed, and the concentration of spermatozoa is readjusted to $3.5 \times 10^6$ motile spermatozoa/ml before being dispersed as 50–100 $\mu$l droplets under paraffin oil. However, valid results can still be obtained using concentrations as low as $1 \times 10^6$ motile spermatozoa/ml (Aitken & Elton, 1986).

The zona-free hamster oocytes, prepared as described by Yanagimachi et al. (1976), are dispensed into the droplets with about 5 oocytes/drop and 20 oocytes/sample.

After a further 3 hours the oocytes are recovered from the droplets, washed free of loosely adherent spermatozoa, compressed to a depth of about 30 $\mu$m under a $22 \times 22$ mm cover slip on a glass slide and assessed for the presence of decondensing sperm heads with an attached or closely associated tail, using phase-contrast microscopy. The number of spermatozoa penetrating each egg is assessed and the results expressed as the mean number of spermatozoa penetrating each oocyte.

### XV.3  Quality control

The assays must be performed with an adequate degree of quality control. The within-assay coefficient of variation should be established by replicating the analysis of a single sample at least 10 times in one assay. Under such circumstances the within-assay coefficient of variation should not exceed 15%. The between-assay coefficient of variation should not exceed 25%; it can be ascertained using a cryostored pool of spermatozoa with a known level of penetration. Any assay in which the value obtained for the standard preparation is more than two standard deviations away from the mean value should be rejected as unreliable. Any analysis in which a penetration score of zero is obtained should be repeated on a separate semen sample.

### References

Aitken, R.J. & Elton, R.A. (1986) Application of a Poisson-gamma model to study the influence of gamete concentration on sperm–oocyte fusion in the zona-free hamster egg penetration test. *Journal of Reproduction and Fertility*, **78**: 733–9.

Aitken, R.J., Templeton, A., Schats, R., Best, F., Richardson, D., Djahanbakhch, O. & Lees, M. (1983) Methods of assessing the functional capacity of human spermatozoa: their role in the selection of patients for in vitro fertilization. In *Fertilization of the Human Egg in vitro*, ed. H. Beier & H. Lindner, pp. 147–65. Berlin: Springer.

Biggers, J.D., Whitten, W.K. & Whittingham, D.G. (1971) The culture of mouse embryos in vitro. In *Methods in Mammalian Embryology*, ed. J.C. Daniel, pp. 86–116. San Francisco: Freeman.

Yanagimachi, R., Yanagimachi, H. & Rogers, B.J. (1976) The use of zona-free animal ova as a test system for the assessment of fertilizing capacity of human spermatozoa. *Biology of Reproduction*, **15**: 471–6.

# Measurement of reactive oxygen species generated by sperm suspensions

## XVI.1 Protocol

This procedure requires the use of a sensitive luminometer (e.g., the Berthold LB 9505) to measure low amounts of light generated by human spermatozoa in the presence of a chemiluminescent probe such as luminol or lucigenin. The methodology described employs a mixture of luminol and horseradish peroxidase to achieve sensitive measurements of hydrogen peroxide generation. However, other probes have also been used to monitor the production of reactive oxygen species (ROS) by the washed human ejaculate including lucigenin which is believed to measure the extracellular release of superoxide anion (Aitken et al., 1992; McKinney et al., 1996).

   (i) Pipette 400 μl of washed human spermatozoa ($10 \times 10^6$ spermatozoa/ml) suspended in a simple Krebs Ringer medium lacking phenol red into a disposable luminometer container being careful to avoid the creation of air bubbles.

   (ii) Add 4 μl of 5-amino-2,3 dehydro-1,4 phthalazinedione (luminol; Sigma Chemical Company, St. Louis, MO) prepared as a 25 mM stock in DMSO (dimethyl sulfoxide), to the container together with 8 μl horseradish peroxidase (12.4 U of horseradish peroxidase Type VI, 310 U/mg: Sigma Chemical Company).

   (iii) Monitor the chemiluminescent signal at 37 °C for about 5 minutes until it has stabilized.

   (iv) FMLP -provocation test for leukocytes

   Add 2 μl of the leukocyte-specific probe formyl-methionyl-leucyl-phenylalanine (FMLP), prepared as a 10 mM stock in DMSO, to the reaction mixture in order to stimulate a chemiluminescent signal from any polymorphs that are present in the sperm suspension (Krausz et al., 1992). Since FMLP receptors are not present on the surface of human spermatozoa, this signal is specific for the leukocyte population and can be calibrated with suspensions containing known numbers of polymorphonuclear leukocytes.

   (v) PMA provocation of ROS generation by leukocytes and spermatozoa

   After the FMLP signal has subsided, treat the sperm suspension with 4 μl phorbol 12-myristate 13-acetate (PMA), prepared as a 1 mM stock solution in DMSO and diluted 1 in 100 to give a 10 μM working stock solution and a final concentration of 100 nM. This

Fig. XVI.1. Patterns of chemiluminescence observed with human sperm suspensions using the luminol-peroxidase system. (*a*) In the presence of leukocyte contamination a burst of ROS generation is observed on addition of the leukocyte-specific probe FMLP (formyl-methionyl-leucyl-phenylalanine). The subsequent addition of PMA (12-myristrate 13-acetate phorbol ester) generates a sustained, intense chemiluminescent signal from both the spermatozoa and leukocyte populations. (*b*) In the absence of leukocyte contamination, the FMLP resonse is lost while PMA elicits a pronounced chemiluminescent signal from the spermatozoa (Krausz et al., 1992).

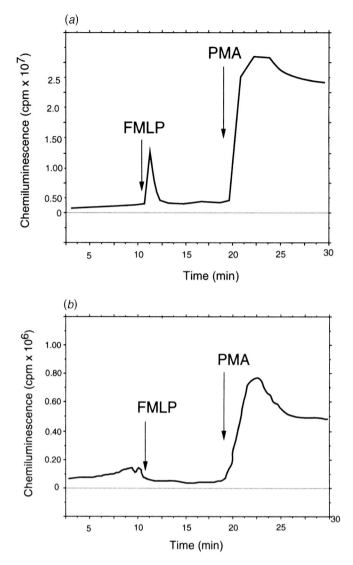

reagent gives an indication of the contributions made by each of the leukocyte and sperm subpopulations to the reactive oxygen generating capacity of the suspension (Fig. XVI.1).

*Note*: The capacity of a leukocyte to generate reactive oxygen species is at least 100 times greater than that of a spermatozoon. A low level of leukocyte contamination can therefore have a major influence on the chemiluminescent signals generated by a sperm suspension.

### References

Aitken, R.J., Buckingham, D.W. & West, K.M. (1992) Reactive oxygen species and human spermatozoa: analysis of the cellular mecha-

nisms involved in luminol- and lucigenin-dependent chemiluminescence. *Journal of Cellular Physiology,* **151**: 466–77.

Krausz, C., West, K, Buckingham, D. & Aitken, R.J. (1992) Analysis of
the interaction between *N*-formylmethionyl-leucyl phenylalanine
and human sperm suspensions: development of a technique for
monitoring the contamination of human semen samples with
leukocytes. *Fertility and Sterility,* **57**: 1317–25.

McKinney, K.A., Lewis, S.E.M. & Thompson, W. (1996) Reactive
oxygen species generation in human sperm: luminol and lucigenin
chemiluminescence probe. *Archives of Andrology,* **36**: 119–25.

# Induced acrosome reaction assay

The acrosome reaction (AR) is an exocytotic process that occurs after the spermatozoa bind to the zona pellucida and must take place before the spermatozoon can penetrate the oocyte vestments and fertilize the oocyte. Calcium influx is believed to be an initiating event in the normal AR. Inducing calcium influx by using a calcium transporting agent, e.g., ionophore A23187, or by progesterone treatment, are ways of testing the competence of capacitated spermatozoa to undergo the AR. However, testing acrosome status needs further evaluation before it can be considered a routine clinical assay.

## XVII.1 Acrosome reaction inducer

Prepare a stock solution of 2–5 mM calcium ionophore A23187 (free acid) in dimethylsulfoxide (DMSO) and store in small aliquots at −20 °C. *Note*: A23187 is light sensitive, so precautions should be taken to prevent exposure to light.

Prepare a working solution by dilution of the stock solution with culture medium such that a small volume (e.g., 2.5–10 µl) may be added to tubes to yield a final concentration of A23187 in the assay of 10 µM and a DMSO concentration of <1%.

## XVII.2 General procedure

(i) Allow 30–60 minutes for complete liquefaction of semen.

(ii) A technique for sperm preparation to obtain a highly motile population free from contaminants such as leukocytes, germ cells, and dead spermatozoa is recommended (see Appendix XVIII) but is not mandatory.

(iii) A bicarbonate-buffered medium, such as BWW (see Appendix XV), Ham's F-10, or synthetic human tubal fluid (HTF), containing 10–35 g/l human serum albumin should be used in the test for culturing the spermatozoa to induce capacitation. Warm the medium before use to 37 °C, preferably in a 5% $CO_2$, 95% air incubator. It is recommended that the capacitation-inducing medium be prepared freshly for each assay.

(iv) Prepare a control and an experimental tube each containing $1 \times 10^6$ motile spermatozoa/ml and incubate for 3 hours to induce capacitation.

(v)     To the experimental tube add a sufficient volume of A23187 working solution to yield a final concentration of $10 \mu M$. To the control tube, add the same volume of DMSO.

(vi)     Incubate both tubes at $37\,°C$ for 15 minutes. Remove a small aliquot from the control and experimental tubes for motility determination before stopping the reaction, e.g., using 3% glutaraldehyde or ethanol.

(vii)     Transfer the fixed spermatozoa to precleaned microscope slides and air dry.

(viii)     Stain the spermatozoa using fluorescent labels evaluated by fluorescence microscopy.

(ix)     Assess the percentage of acrosome-reacted spermatozoa in the experimental samples (test % AR) and the control samples (control % AR).

## XVII.3 Results

The acrosome reaction after ionophore challenge (ARIC) is the test % AR minus the control % AR. The normal value is 15%. Values $<10\%$ are considered abnormal. Values between 10% and 15% suggest that sperm function may be abnormal. If $>20\%$ of spermatozoa in the control tube show a spontaneous AR after 3 hours' incubation then premature AR has occurred.

## XVII.4 Quality control

A positive control sample must be run each time the test is performed. To ensure that each new preparation of stain has been made properly, a crossover test should be performed with the old stain using positive control spermatozoa with a known response.

### Reference

European Society of Human Reproduction and Embryology (1996) Consensus workshop on advanced diagnostic andrology. *Human Reproduction*, **11**: 1463–79.

# Sperm preparation techniques

**XVIII.1** **Procedures**

Several simple preparation techniques are described. For all of them the culture medium suggested is supplemented Earle's balanced salt solution, although other media that will support sperm motility and viability for at least 18 hours at 37 °C may be used, e.g., Ham's F10, Human tubal fluid (HTF).

**XVIII.2** **Swim-up**

Supplemented Earle's medium (1.2 ml) is gently layered over semen (1 ml) in a sterile 15 ml conical-based centrifuge tube. The tube is inclined at an angle of 45° and incubated for 1 hour at 37 °C. It is then gently returned to the upright position and the uppermost 1 ml removed. This aliquot of motile cells is then diluted with eight volumes of supplemented Earle's, centrifuged at 500$g$ for 5 minutes, and finally resuspended in 0.5 ml of Earle's medium for the assessment of sperm concentration or sperm function, or for other procedures.

*Constituents of supplemented Earle's medium*

---

46 ml Earle's balanced salt solution
4 ml heat-inactivated (56 °C for 20 minutes) patient's serum
1.5 mg sodium pyruvate
0.18 ml sodium lactate (60% syrup)
100 mg sodium bicarbonate

---

or

---

50 ml Earle's balanced salt solution
300 mg human serum albumin[a]
1.5 mg sodium pyruvate
0.18 ml sodium lactate (60% syrup)
100 mg sodium bicarbonate

---

[a] For assisted reproduction procedures such as in vitro fertilization (IVF), artificial insemination, or gamete intrafallopian transfer, it is imperative that the human serum albumin be highly purified and free from viral, bacterial, and prion contamination. Some preparations of albumin have been designed for such procedures (e.g., from Irvine Scientific, Santa Ana, CA, USA; Armour Pharmaceuticals, Eastbourne, United Kingdom).

## XVIII.3  Discontinuous density gradients

(i)   Pipette 3 ml of 80% Percoll or alternative product into a 15 ml sterile conical-bottomed tube.

(ii)  Gently pipette 3 ml of 40% Percoll or alternative product on top of the 80% layer, taking care not to disturb the interface between the two layers.

(iii) Gently layer 1–2 ml semen over the gradient and centrifuge at $500g$ for 20 minutes.

(iv)  Resuspended the pellet at the bottom of the 80% fraction in 5–10 ml of Earle's medium and centrifuge at $500g$ for 5 minutes before resuspending it in 1 ml of Earle's medium.

(v)   Estimate the sperm concentration and motility or sperm function.

It should be noted that Percoll has been withdrawn from use in human clinical applications and can now be used only for research purposes. However, other products are available for human clinical applications, e.g., PureSperm (NidaCon Labs, Gothenburg, Sweden) or Isolate (Irvine Scientific, NidaCon, Santa Ana, CA, USA). To date, only the manufacturer's instructions for these techniques are available. There are few publications comparing their efficiency to that of other density gradient centrifugation techniques although some clinics have found the techniques to be equal to those useing Percoll (Perez et al., 1997). Both PureSperm and Isolate are isotonic; thus volumetric dilutions (8 + 2 and 4 + 6) are required. PureSperm is in a Hepes-buffered medium; gradients should thus be made using a Hepes-buffered medium.

*Constituents of isotonic Percoll or alternative product*

10 ml of 10x concentrated Earle's medium (e.g., from Flow Laboratories)
90 ml density gradient material
300 mg human serum albumin
3 mg sodium pyruvate
0.37 ml sodium lactate (60% syrup)
200 mg sodium bicarbonate

*Constituents of 80% density gradient material*

40 ml isotonic material
10 ml supplemented Earle's medium

*Constituents of 40% density gradient material*

20 ml isotonic material
30 ml supplemented Earle's medium

### XVIII.4 Preparation of poor quality samples

In cases of severe oligozoospermia and/or asthenozoospermia, density gradients are preferable to the 'swim-up' method because of the improved recoveries obtained. Moreover the scale and composition of the gradient can be altered to meet the specific needs of individual samples. One possibility, for example, is to apply the sample to several minidensity gradients (Mortimer, 1994b) containing only 0.3 ml volumes of the 40% and 80% density gradient material.

### References

Mortimer, D. (1994b) *Practical Laboratory Andrology.* p.393. Oxford: Oxford University Press.

Perez, S.M., Chan, P.J., Patton, W.C. & King, A. (1997). Silane-coated silica particle colloid processing of human sperm. *Journal of Assisted Reproduction and Genetics,* **14**: 388–93.

# Quality control (QC) procedures

### XIX.1 QC test samples

QC specimens should be representative of the range of semen samples processed in the laboratory. If only a small number of QC samples are to be analysed, those with results in clinically significant ranges (concentration $5 \times 10^6$–$30 \times 10^6$/ml, motility 10–40%, and normal morphology below 20%) should be chosen. Centres supplying QC samples for assessment by others need to ensure that they are negative for hepatitis and HIV.

### XIX.2 Materials for quality control

Aliquots of pooled semen samples can be stored frozen or liquid with a preservative (10% formalin, 100 $\mu$l per ml of semen) at 4°C and analysed at intervals for sperm concentration. Cryopreserved pooled semen may also be used for QC of motility. Videotapes can be used for sperm motility and photographs, video tapes and stained or unstained fixed smears on slides can be used for sperm morphology. However, some problems with these materials should be recognized. Mixing of pooled semen may be incomplete, especially before or after thawing. Video tapes are particularly useful for training in motility and morphology assessment. However, their use for QC tends to give an optimistic impression and they should not be used to the exclusion of replicate assessments of semen specimens. Stained slides for sperm morphology tend to fade, and prefixed smears tend to deteriorate. Spermatozoa may not survive cryopreservation sufficiently well to be a useful source of internal and external QC materials for motility and sperm antibody tests. Sperm antibody positive serum may be used for QC of indirect immunobead tests but is suboptimal for direct immunobead tests. Thus QC practice where the same QC pools are included in every assay, is not always feasible.

### XIX.3 Calibration of equipment

Pipettes can be calibrated by weighing distilled water from single or multiple transfers with replication to allow both accuracy and precision to be determined. It is necessary to correct for the temperature effect on the density of water, i.e., at 20°C 1 ml of distilled water weighs 0.9982 g. Alternatively, micropipettes may be calibrated by diluting a coloured substance that can be measured accurately with a spectrophotometer. Counting chambers can be calibrated with bead suspensions of known particle density. Counting chamber depths can be determined with a Vernier scale on the fine focus of a microscope by focusing on the grid and then on an ink mark on the underside of the cover slip. Measurements should be repeated a number of times, e.g., ten times. Results should agree with the stated volume or depth within the error of the measurements ($\pm 2SD$). Balances should be checked regularly with internal calibrators and by external calibration at the time of regular laboratory maintenance service. Temperatures of incubators and warm stages should be checked with thermometers which are in turn calibrated regularly. Gas mixtures should be checked daily with the incubator readout, by Fyrite or other systems weekly to monthly, and by gas sampling at the time of servicing. Other laboratory equipment and reagents such as pH meters should also be checked with standards at 3- to 6-month intervals.

## XIX.4  Some external quality assessment schemes

| | |
|---|---|
| AUSTRALASIA<br>Fertility Society of Australia<br>External Quality Assurance Schemes<br>    for Reproductive Medicine<br>PO Box 1101<br>West Leederville<br>Western Australia 6901, Australia | EUROPE<br>UKNEQAS Schemes for Andrology<br>Department of Reproductive<br>    Medicine<br>St. Mary's Hospital<br>Whitworth Park<br>Manchester M13 0JH, United<br>    Kingdom |
| SCANDINAVIA<br>NAFA (Nordic Association for<br>    Andrology)<br>Andrology Unit,<br>Reproductive Medicine Centre<br>Karolinska Hospital<br>PO Box 140<br>SE-171 76 Stockholm, Sweden | USA<br>American Association of<br>    Bioanalysts<br>Proficiency Testing Service,<br>205 West Levee<br>Brownsville,<br>Texas 78520-5596, USA |

*Notes:*
National external quality control programmes have been created in Belgium, the Netherlands and France, and are being developed in other countries.

### References

Altman, D.G. (1991) *Practical Statistics for Medical Research*. London: Chapman and Hall.

Barnett, R.N. (1979) *Clinical Laboratory Statistics*, 2nd ed. Boston: Little, Brown.

# Sample Record Form for Cervical Mucus Scoring and Postcoital Test

Date of last menstrual period

Day   Month   Year

Daily cervical mucus score

| | Day Month | Day Month | Day Month | Day Month |
|---|---|---|---|---|
| Date | | | | |
| Day of cycle | | | | |
| Volume | | | | |
| Consistency | | | | |
| Ferning | | | | |
| Spinnbarkeit | | | | |
| Cellularity | | | | |
| Total score | | | | |
| pH | | | | |

Postcoital test

Day   Month

Date

Time after coitus (h)

| | Vaginal pool | Endocervical pool |
|---|---|---|
| Spermatozoa/mm³ | | |

Motility (% spermatozoa)

| | | |
|---|---|---|
| (a) Rapid progression | | |
| (b) Slow progression | | |
| (c) Nonprogressive | | |
| (d) Immotile | | |

# Sperm–cervical mucus interaction: the capillary tube test

The capillary tube test was originally designed by Kremer (1965). It measures the ability of spermatozoa to penetrate a column of cervical mucus in a capillary tube. Various modifications of capillary tube tests have been proposed. The procedure recommended here is based on the original test developed by Kremer, which most clinicians have adopted.

### XXI.1 Equipment

Various types of capillary tubes have been used but flat capillary tubes, 5 cm long and 3 mm wide by 0.3 mm deep in cross section are recommended. Such tubes can be obtained from Camlab Ltd., Cambridge, United Kingdom.

The Kremer sperm penetration meter (Fig. XXI.1) may be constructed in the laboratory as follows:

(i) Glue onto a glass slide three reservoirs (R) of semicircular cross-section (radius about 3.5 mm).

(ii) A second glass slide is then glued onto the first. The second slide is 1.5 cm shorter and is positioned at a distance of 5 mm from the reservoirs. This construction prevents creeping of the seminal fluid between the capillary tube and the glass slide. A centimetre scale is present on the slides.

### XXI.2 Method

Fresh semen, not older than 1 hour after ejaculation, should be used. Cervical mucus is aspirated into a capillary tube, making sure that no air bubbles are introduced. One end of the tube is sealed with plasticine, modelling clay, or similar agents. Enough sealer should be applied that the mucus column protrudes slightly out of the open end of the tube. The open end of the capillary tube is then placed on a slide so that it projects about 0.5 cm into the reservoir containing the semen sample. During the process of sperm penetration, the slide should be placed in a covered Petri dish with damp sponge on the sides, to maintain humidity and prevent drying of the semen and mucus. The measurements are carried out preferably in a chamber with an ambient temperature of 37 °C.

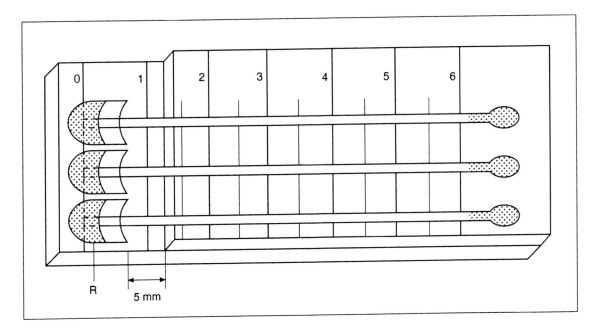

Fig. XXI.1. The Kremer sperm
penetration meter (see text).

### XXI.3 Assessment of the test

After 2 hours, the migration distance, penetration density, migration reduction, and presence of spermatozoa with forward motility are read.

The capillary tubes may be inspected again after 24 hours for the presence of forward moving spermatozoa only.

Variables to be assessed after two hours are defined as follows.

*XXI.3.1 Migration distance*

The distance from the end of the capillary tube in the semen reservoir to the foremost spermatozoon in the tube.

*XXI.3.2 Penetration density*

This is determined at distances of 1 and 4.5 cm from the end of the capillary tube in the semen reservoir. At each distance the mean number of spermatozoa per low power field (LPF; $10 \times 10$) is determined. The mean number is obtained from estimations of five adjacent low power fields. The mean of the estimations is expressed in one of the penetration density classes (see Table XXI.1). For the classification of the test, the highest penetration density class is recorded.

Table XXI.1. *Order of classes of penetration density*

| Penetration density class | Rank order |
|---|---|
| 0 | 1 |
| 0–5 | 2 |
| 6–10 | 3 |
| 11–20 | 4 |
| 21–50 | 5 |
| 51–100 | 6 |
| >100 | 7 |

### XXI.3.3 Migration reduction

This indicates the *decrease* in penetration density at 4.5 cm compared to the penetration density at 1 cm. It is expressed as the difference in rank order number.

*Examples*

1. Penetration density at 1 cm is 51–100 and at 4.5 cm is 6–10. The migration reduction value is 3 (rank order 6 to rank order 3; Table XXI.1).

2. Penetration density at 1 cm is 21–50 and at 4.5 cm is 51–100. The migration reduction value is zero because there is no decrease in penetration density.

### XXI.3.4 Duration of progressive movements

The presence in the cervical mucus of spermatozoa with forward motility may be determined after 2 and 24 hours.
The results are classified according to Table XXI.2.

Table XXI.2. *Classification of the test results*

| Migration distance (cm) | Penetration density (spermatozoa per low power field) | Migration reduction from 1 to 4.5 cm (decrease in rank order number) | Duration of progressive movements in cervical mucus (hours) | Classification |
|---|---|---|---|---|
| 1 | 0 | — | — | Negative |
| <3 or | <10 or | >3 or | 2 | Poor |
| | All combinations of test results that cannot be classified as: negative, poor or good | | | Fair |
| 4.5 and | >50 and | <3 and | >24 | Good |

112

## Reference

Kremer, J. (1965) A simple penetration test. *International Journal of Fertility*, **10**: 209–15.

# Basic requirements for an andrology laboratory

The following is a list of the supplies and equipment that would enable a laboratory to function as an andrology laboratory and to perform the basic tests suggested in this manual. This assumes that a refrigerator, a centrifuge (swing-out rotor), and an incubator are already available.

### A. Safety in the andrology laboratory
1. Rubber gloves
2. Face masks
3. Laboratory coats
4. Sodium hypochlorite, 5.25 g/l (e.g., household bleach diluted 1:10 with water)
5. Protective safety glasses
6. First-aid kit
7. Eye-washing solution
8. Shower (optional)
9. Container for sharp objects

### B. Semen analysis
1. *WHO Laboratory Manual for the Examination of Human Semen and Sperm- Cervical Mucus Interaction* (fourth edition)
2. Record forms for semen analysis
3. Wide-mouth disposable containers with lids. These should be demonstrated not to have toxic effects on spermatozoa as follows:
   (i) select semen samples with high sperm concentration and good sperm motility;
   (ii) divide each sample and put half in a glass container known to be non-toxic (control) and the other half in the test container;
   (iii) assess sperm motility and vitality at hourly intervals for 4 hours;
   (iv) repeat (i) – (iii) for several samples. If there are no differences between control and test assessments, the test containers are considered to be nontoxic.
4. Pasteur pipettes with latex droppers or plastic disposable transfer pipettes
5. Automatic pipettes (e.g., Eppendorf, Oxford, Finnpipet, Pipetman, available from many suppliers)

6. Positive displacement pipette to measure 50 µl, such as the Wiretrol II W-100 (Drummond Scientific Co., 500 Parkway, Broomhall, PA 19008, USA), the Gilson pipette, (Gilson Medical Electronics SA, F-95400, Villiers le Bel, France); and the SMI Digital Adjust Micro/Pettor Model P5068-20D for volumes of 20 µl to 100 µl (SMI Liquid Handling Products, American Hospital Supply Corporation, Miami, FL 33152, USA)

7. Laboratory counter, such as the Clay Adams Lab Counter (Fisher Scientific, Springfield, NJ, USA, catalogue No. 02-670-13) and the 'Assistant' (Karl Willers, Laborbedarf D48151 Münster, Germany).

8. Haemocytometers (improved Neubauer)

9. Warming plate (bench top)

10. Vortex mixer

11. Phase-contrast microscope, to include ×10, ×20, ×40 phase objectives, ×100 oil-immersion objective, and ×10 (wide-field) eyepiece. The microscope should be checked regularly to ensure that the phase rings are adjusted for optimal use.

12. 50-watt light source

13. Microscope slides

14. Appropriate quality control

### C. Sperm–cervical mucus interaction

1. Record forms for scoring

2. Mucus sampling syringe, e.g., Aspiglaire (BICEF, L'Aigle, France)

3. Glass capillary tubes for the capillary tube test, 3 mm wide, 0.3 mm deep, 5 cm long (Camlab Ltd. Cambridge, United Kingdom).

### D. Reagents for Immunobead or MAR test
See Appendices VIII and IX

### E. Reagents for sperm morphology
See Appendices III to VII.

### F. Graphs
Figs. 2.3 and 2.6 of this manual for display in the laboratory.

Fig. 2.3. Approximate 95% confidence interval ranges for differences between two percentages determined from duplicate counts of 100, 200 or 400 spermatozoa. To assess the percentages from two counts of 200, calculate their average and difference. If the difference is greater than indicated by the $N = 200$ curve, the sample must be reanalysed. The lower curve shows the increase in precision for two assessments of 400 spermatozoa ($N = 400$). For an average result of 5%, the 95% confidence interval is 3%. The large statistical counting errors associated with counting only 100 spermatozoa are apparent from the top curve ($N = 100$). For a result of 5%, the two single assessments of 100 spermatozoa could be 3% and 9% by chance alone.

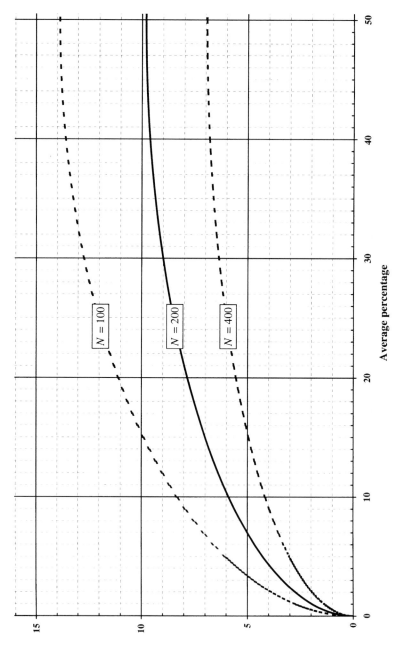

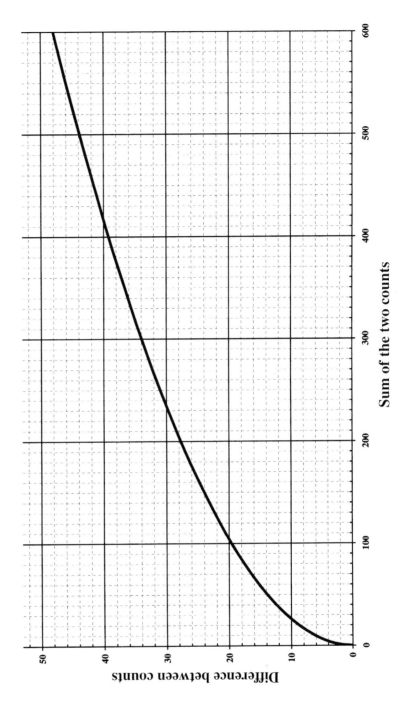

Fig. 2.6. Approximate 95% confidence interval for differences between two counts. To assess these counts, calculate their sum and difference. If the difference is greater than indicated by the curve there may be a systematic error (see Chapter 4) and the sample must be reanalysed. The large statistical counting errors associated with counting fewer than 200 spermatozoa are apparent. For example, for a mean count of 60 spermatozoa (sum 120), the two counts could be 50 and 70 by chance alone.

# Bibliography

*Asterisk indicates review article*

Aitken, R.J. & Clarkson, J.S. (1987) Cellular basis of defective sperm function and its association with genesis of reactive oxygen species by human spermatozoa. *Journal of Reproduction and Fertility*, **81**: 459–69.

Aitken, R.J. & West, K.M. (1990) Analysis of the relationship between reactive oxygen species production and leucocyte infiltration in fractions of human semen separated on Percoll gradients. *International Journal of Andrology*, **13**: 433–51.

Aitken, R.J. & Brindle, J.P. (1993) Analysis of the ability of three probes targeting the outer acrosomal membrane or acrosomal contents to detect the acrosome reaction in human spermatozoa. *Human Reproduction*, **8**: 1663–9.

Aitken, R.J., Buckingham, D.W. & Huang, G.F. (1993) Analysis of the response of human spermatozoa to A23187 employing a novel technique for assessing the acrosome reaction. *Journal of Andrology*, **14**: 132–41.

Aitken, R.J., Buckingham, D.W., Harkiss, D., Paterson, M., Fisher, H. & Irvine, D.S. (1996) The extragenomic action of progesterone on human spermatozoa is influenced by redox regulated changes in tyrosine phosphorylation during capacitation. *Molecular and Cellular Endocrinology*, **117**: 83–93.

Altman, D.G. (1991) *Practical Statistics for Medical Research*. London: Chapman and Hall.

Alvarez, J.G., Touchstone, J.C., Blasco, L. & Storey, B.T. (1987) Spontaneous lipid peroxidation and production of hydrogen peroxide and superoxide in human spermatozoa. Superoxide dismutase as major enzyme protectant against oxygen toxicity. *Journal of Andrology*, **8**: 338–48.

Ayvaliotis, B., Bronson, R., Rosenfeld, D. & Cooper, G. (1985) Conception rates in couples where autoimmunity to sperm is detected. *Fertility and Sterility*, **43**: 739–42.

Aziz, N., Buchan, I., Taylor, C., Kingland. C.R. & Lewis-Jones, I. (1996) The sperm deformity index: a reliable predictor of the outcome of oocyte fertilization in vitro. *Fertility and Sterility*, **66**: 1000-8.

Barnett, R.N. (1979) *Clinical Laboratory Statistics*, 2nd ed. Boston: Little, Brown.

Barratt, C.L.R., Dunphy, B.C., McLeod, I. & Cooke, I.D. (1992) The poor prognostic value of low to moderate levels of sperm surface bound antibodies. *Human Reproduction*, **7**: 95–8.

Barratt, C.L.R., Tomlinson, M.J. & Cooke, I.D. (1993) Prospective study of leukocytes and leukocyte subpopulations in semen suggests they are not a cause of male infertility. *Fertility and Sterility*, **60**: 1069–75.

Blackmore, P.F., Beebe, S.J., Danforth, D.R. & Alexander, N. (1990) Progesterone and 17-hydroxyprogesterone: novel stimulators of calcium influx in human sperm. *Journal of Biological Chemistry*, **265**: 1376–80.

Bland, J.M. & Altman, D.G. (1986) Statistical methods for assessing agreement between two methods of clinical measurement. *Lancet*, **i**: 307–10.

Bronson, R.A., Cooper, G.W. & Rosenfeld, D. (1982) Detection of sperm specific antibodies on the spermatozoa surface by immunobead binding. *Archives of Andrology*, **9**: 61.

*Bronson, R.A., Cooper, G.W. & Rosenfeld, D. (1984) Sperm antibodies: their role in infertility. *Fertility and Sterility*, **42**: 171–83.

Burkman, L.J., Kruger, T.F., Coddington, C.C., Rosenwaks, Z., Franken, D.R. & Hodgen, G.D. (1988) The hemizona assay (HZA): development of a diagnostic test for the binding of human spermatozoa to human hemizona pellucida to predict fertilization potential. *Fertility and Sterility*, **49**: 688–97.

Canale, D., Giorgi, M., Gasperini, M., Pucci, E., Barletta, D., Gasperi, M. & Martino, E. (1994) Inter and intra-individual variability of sperm morphology after selection with three different techniques: layering, swimup from pellet and Percoll. *Journal of Endocrinological Investigation*, **17**: 729–32.

Clarke, G.N., Stojanoff, A. & Cauchi, M.N. (1982) Immunoglobulin class of sperm-bound antibodies in semen. In *Immunology of Reproduction*, ed. K. Bratanov, pp. 482–5. Sofia, Bulgaria: Bulgarian Academy of Sciences Pres.

Clarke, G.N., Elliott, P.J. & Smaila, C. (1985) Detection of sperm antibodies in semen using the Immunobead test: a survey of 813 consecutive patients. *American Journal of Reproductive Immunology and Microbiology*, **7**: 118–23.

Clements, S., Cooke, I.D. & Barratt, C.L.R. (1995) Implementing comprehensive quality control in the andrology laboratory. *Human Reproduction*, **10**: 2096–106.

Comhaire, F., Verschraegen, G. & Vermeulen, L. (1980) Diagnosis of accessory gland infection and its possible role in male infertility. *International Journal of Andrology*, **3**: 32–45.

Cooper, T.G., Yeung, C.H., Nashan, D., Jockenhövel, F. & Nieschlag, E. (1990) Improvement in the assessment of human epididymal function by the use of inhibitors in the assay of $\alpha$-glucosidase in seminal plasma. *International Journal of Andrology*, **13**: 297–305.

Cooper, T.G., Neuwinger, J., Bahrs, S. & Nieschlag, E. (1992) Internal quality control of semen analysis. *Fertility and Sterility*, **58**: 172–8.

*Cross, N.L. (1995) Methods for evaluating the acrosomal status of human sperm. In *Human Sperm Acrosome Reaction*, ed. P. Fenichel & J. Parinaud, pp. 277–85. (Colloques INSERM) John Libbey Eurotext.

Cross, N.L., Morales, P., Overstreet, J.W. & Hanson, F.W. (1986) Two simple methods for detecting acrosome-reacted human sperm. *Gamete Research*, **15**: 213–26.

Cummins, J.M., Pember, S.M., Jequier, A.M., Yovich, J.L. & Hartmann, P.E. (1991) A test of the human sperm acrosome reaction following ionophore challenge: relationship to fertility and other seminal parameters. *Journal of Andrology*, **12**: 98–103.

*Davis, R.O. & Katz, D.F. (1992) Standardization and comparability of CASA instruments. *Journal of Andrology*, **13**: 81–6.

Davis, R.O. & Gravance, C.G. (1993) Standardization of specimen preparation, staining and sampling methods improves automated sperm-head morphometry analysis. *Fertility and Sterility*, **59**: 412–17.

*De Jonge, C.J. (1994) The diagnostic significance of the induced acrosome reaction. *Reproductive Medicine Review*, **3**: 159–78.

Drevius, L. & Eriksson, H. (1966) Osmotic swelling of mammalian spermatozoa. *Experimental Cell Research*, **42**: 136–56.

Drobnis, E.Z., Yudin, A.L., Cherr, G.N. & Katz, D.F. (1988) Hamster sperm penetration of the zona pellucida: kinematic analysis and mechanical implications. *Developmental Biology*, **130**: 311–23.

Dunphy, B.C., Kay R., Barratt, C.L.R. & Cooke, I.D. (1989) Quality control during the conventional analysis of semen, an essential exercise. *Journal of Andrology*, **10**: 378–85.

Eggert-Kruse, W., Leinhos, G., Gerhard, I. Tilgen, W. & Runnebaum, B. (1989) Prognostic value of in vitro sperm penetration into hormonally standardized human cervical mucus. *Fertility and Sterility*, **51**: 317–23.

Eggert-Kruse, W., Köhler, A., Rohr, G. & Runnebaum, B. (1993) The pH as an important determinant of sperm-mucus interaction. *Fertility and Sterility*, **59**: 617–28.

*Eliasson, R. (1971) Standards for investigation of human semen. *Andrologia*, **3**: 49–64.

*Eliasson, R. (1981) Analysis of semen. In: Burger, H. & de Kretser, D. ed. *The Testis*, New York, Raven Press, pp. 381–99.

Enginsu, M.E., Dumoulin, C.J.M., Pieters, M.H.E.C., Bras, M., Evers, J.L.H. & Geraedts, J.P.M. (1991) Evaluation of human sperm morphology using strict criteria after Diff-Quik staining: correlation of morphology with fertilization in vitro. *Human Reproduction*, **6**: 854–8.

European Society of Human Reproduction and Embryology (1996) Consensus workshop on advanced diagnostic andrology techniques. *Human Reproduction*, **11**: 1463–79.

Fenichel, P., Hsi, B.L., Farahifar, D., Donzeau, M., Barrier-Delpech, D. & Yehy, C.J. (1989) Evaluation of the human sperm acrosome reaction using a mono-clonal antibody, GB24, and fluorescence activated cell sorter. *Journal of Reproduction and Fertility*, **87**: 699–706.

Franken, D.R., Oehinger, S., Burkman, L.J., Coddington, C.C., Kruger, T.F., Rosenwaks, Z., Acosta, A.A. & Hodgen, G.D. (1989) The hemizona assay (HZA): a predictor of human sperm fertilizing potential in in vitro fertiliza-tion (IVF) treatment. *Journal of In Vitro Fertilization and Embryo Transfer*, **6**: 44–50.

Fredricsson, B. & Bjork, R. (1977) Morphology of postcoital spermatozoa in the cervical secretion and its clinical significance. *Fertility and Sterility*, **28**: 841–5.

Garrett, C. & Baker, H.W.G. (1995) A new fully automated system for the mor-phometric analysis of human sperm heads. *Fertility and Sterility*, **63**: 1306–17.

Garrett, C., Liu, D.Y. & Baker, H.W.G. (1997) Selectivity of the human sperm-zona pellucida binding process to sperm head morphometry. *Fertility and Sterility*, **67**, 362–71.

Gellert-Mortimer, S.T., Clarke, G.N., Baker, H.W.G., Hyne, R.V. & Johnson, W.I.H. (1988) Evaluation of Nycodenz and Percoll density gradients for the selection of motile human spermatozoa. *Fertility and Sterility*, **49**: 335–41.

Ginsberg, K.A. & Armant, D.R. (1990) The influence of chamber characteristics on the reliability of sperm concentration and movement measurements obtained by manual and videomicrographic analysis. *Fertility and Sterility*, **53**: 882–7.

Gomez, E., Buckingham, D.W., Brindle, J., Lanzafame, F., Irvine, D.S. & Aitken, R.J. (1996) Development of an image analysis system to monitor the retention of residual cytoplasm by human spermatozoa: correlation with biochemical markers of the cytoplasmic space, oxidative stress, and sperm function. *Journal of Andrology*, **17**: 276–87.

*Griveau, J.F. & LeLannou, D. (1997) Reactive oxygen species and human spermatozoa: physiology and pathology. *International Journal of Andrology*, **20**: 61–9.

Gruber, W. & Möllering, H. (1966) Determination of citrate with citrate lyase. *Analytical Biochemistry*, **17**: 369–76.

Heite, H. -J. & Wetterauer, W. (1979) Acid phosphatase in seminal fluid: method of estimation and diagnostic significance. *Andrologia*, **11**: 113–22.

Hellstrom, W.J.G., Samuels, S.J., Waits, A.B. & Overstreet J.W. (1989) A comparison of the usefulness of SpermMar and Immunobead tests for the detection of antisperm antibodies. *Fertility and Sterility*, **52**: 1027–31.

Henley, N., Baron, C. & Roberts, K.D. (1994) Flow cytometric evaluation of the acrosome reaction of human spermatozoa: a new method using a photoactivated supravital stain. *International Journal of Andrology*, **17**: 78–84.

Insler, V., Melmed, H., Eichenbrenner, I., Serr, D.M. & Lunnenfeld, B. (1972) The cervical score. A simple semiquantitative method for monitoring of the menstrual cycle. *International Journal of Gynaecology and Obstetrics*, **10**: 223–8.

Irvine, D.S., Macleod, I.C., Templeton, A.A., Masterton, A. & Taylor, A. (1994) A prospective clinical study of the relationship between the computer-assisted assessment of human semen quality and the achievement of pregnancy in vivo. *Human Reproduction*, **9**: 2324–34.

Iwasaki, A. & Gagnon, C. (1992) Formation of reactive oxygen species in spermatozoa of infertile patients. *Fertility and Sterility*, **57**: 2409–16.

Jeyendran, R.S., Van der Ven, H.H., Perez-Pelaez, M. Crabo, B.G. & Zaneveld, L.J.D. (1984) Development of an assay to assess the functional integrity of the human sperm membrane and its relationship to the other semen characteristics. *Journal of Reproduction and Fertility*, **70**: 219–28.

Johnson, D.E., Confino, E. & Jeyendran, R.S. (1996) Glass wool column filtration versus mini-Percoll gradient for processing poor quality semen samples. *Fertility and Sterility*, **66**: 459–62.

Jones, R., Mann, T. & Sherins, R. (1979) Peroxidative breakdown of phospholipids by human spermatozoa, spermicidal properties of fatty acid peroxides and protective action of seminal plasma. *Fertility and Sterility*, **31**: 531–7.

Jouannet, P., Ducot, B., Feneux, D. & Spira, A. (1988) Male factors and the likelihood of pregnancy in infertile couples. I. Study of sperm characteristics. *International Journal of Andrology*, **11**: 379–94.

Katz, D.F., Overstreet, J.W., Samuels, S.J., Niswander, P.W., Bloom, T.D. & Lewis, E.L. (1986) Morphometric analysis of spermatozoa in the assessment of human male fertility. *Journal of Andrology*, **7**: 203–10.

Knuth, U.A., Neuwinger, J. & Nieschlag, E. (1989) Bias of routine semen analysis by uncontrolled changes in laboratory environment: detection by long term sampling of monthly means for quality control. *International Journal of Andrology*, **12**: 375–83.

Kobayashi, T., Jinno, M., Sugimura, K., Nozawa, S., Sugiyama, T. & Lida, E. (1991). Sperm morphological assessment based on strict criteria and in vitro fertilization outcome. *Human Reproduction*, **6**: 983–6.

Krause, W. (1995) Computer-assisted sperm analysis system: comparison with routine evaluation and prognostic value in male fertility and assisted reproduction. *Human Reproduction*, **10**: suppl. 1, 60–6.

Kremer, J. & Jager, S. (1980) Characteristics of anti-spermatozoal antibodies responsible for the shaking phenomenon, with special regard to immunoglobulin class and antigen-reactive sites. *International Journal of Andrology*, **3**: 143–52.

Kruger, T.F., Menkveld, R., Stander, F.S.H., Lombard, C.J., Van der Merwe, J.P., Van

Zyl, J.A. & Smith, K. (1986). Sperm morphologic features as a prognostic factor in in vitro fertilization. *Fertility and Sterility*, **46**: 1118–23.

Kruger, T.F., Ackerman, S.B., Simmons, K.F., Swanson, R.J., Brugo, S.S. & Acosta, A.A. (1987) A quick, reliable staining technique for human sperm morphology. *Archives of Andrology*, **18**: 275–7.

Kruger, T.F., Acosta, A.A., Simmons, K.F., Swanson, R.J., Matta, J.F. & Oehninger, S. (1988) Predictive value of abnormal sperm morphology in in vitro fertilization. *Fertility and Sterility*, **49**: 112–17.

Kruger, T.F., Oehninger, S., Franken, D.R., & Hodgen, G.D. (1991) Hemizona assay: use of fresh versus salt-stored human oocytes to evaluate sperm binding potential to the zona pellucida. *Journal of In-vitro Fertilization and Embryo Transfer*, **8**: 154–6.

Kruger, T.F., Franken, D.R. & Menkveld, R. (1993) *The Self Teaching Programme for Strict Sperm Morphology*. Bellville, South Africa: MQ Medical.

Kruger, T.F., du Toit, T.C., Franken, D.R., Menkveld, R. & Lombard, C.J. (1995) Sperm morphology: assessing the agreement between the manual method (strict criteria) and the sperm morphology analyzer IVOS. *Fertility and Sterility*, **63**: 134–41.

Kruger, T.F., Lacquet, F.A., Sarmiento, C.A.S., Menkveld, R., Ozgur, K., Lombard, C.J. & Franken, D.R. (1996) A prospective study on the predictive value of normal sperm morphology evaluated by computer (IVOS) *Fertility and Sterility*, **66**: 285–91.

Liu, D.Y. & Baker, H.W.G. (1992) Morphology of spermatozoa bound to the zona pellucida of human oocytes that failed to fertilize in vitro. *Journal of Reproduction and Fertility*, **94**: 71–84.

Liu, D.Y., Lopata, A., Johnston, W.I.H. & Baker, H.W.G. (1988) A human sperm-zona pellucida binding test using oocytes that failed to fertilize in-vitro. *Fertility and Sterility*, **50**: 782–8.

Liu, D.Y., Clarke, G.Y., Lopata, A., Johnson, W.I.H. & Baker, H.W.G. (1989) A sperm-zona pellucida binding test and *in-vitro* fertilization. *Fertility and Sterility*, **52**: 281–7.

Makler, A. (1980). The improved ten-micrometer chamber for rapid sperm count and motility evaluation. *Fertility and Sterility*, **33**: 337–8.

Matson, P.L. (1995) External quality control assessment for semen analysis and sperm antibody detection: results of a pilot scheme. *Human Reproduction*, **10**: 620–5.

Meares, E.M. & Stamey, T.A. (1972) The diagnosis and management of bacterial prostatitis. *British Journal of Urology*, **44**: 175–9.

Menkveld, R. & Kruger, T.F. (1996). Evaluation of sperm morphology by light microscopy. In *Human Spermatozoa in Assisted Reproduction*, ed. A.A. Acosta & T.F. Kruger, pp. 89–107, 2nd ed. Parthenon Publishing Group.

Menkveld, R., Stander, F.S.H., Kotze, T.J.V.W., Kruger, T.F. & van Zyl, J.A. (1990) The evaluation of morphological characteristics of human spermatozoa according to stricter criteria. *Human Reproduction*, **5**: 586–92.

Meschede, D., Keck, C., Zander, M., Cooper T.G., Yeung, C.H. & Nieschlag, E. (1993) Influence of three different preparation techniques on the results of human sperm morphology analysis. *International Journal of Andrology*, **16**: 362–9.

Moghissi, K.S. (1976) Post-coital test: physiological basis, technique and interpretation. *Fertility and Sterility*, **27**: 117–29.

*Mortimer D. (1994a) Laboratory standards in routine clinical andrology. *Reproductive Medicine Review*, **3**: 97–111.

*Mortimer D. (1994b) *Practical Laboratory Andrology*. Oxford, Oxford University Press.

Mortimer, D., Leslie, E.E., Kelly, R.W. & Templeton, A.A. (1982) Morphological selection of human spermatozoa in vivo and in vitro. *Journal of Reproduction and Fertility*, **64**: 391–9.

Mortimer, D., Shu, M.A. & Tan, R. (1986) Standardization and quality control of sperm concentration and sperm motility counts in semen analysis. *Human Reproduction*, **1**: 299–303.

Mortimer, D., Shu, M.A., Tan, R. & Mortimer, S.T. (1989) A technical note on diluting semen for the haemocytometric determination of sperm concentration. *Human Reproduction*, **4**: 166–8.

Mortimer, D., Mortimer, S.T., Shu, M.A. & Swart, R. (1990) A simplified approach to sperm–cervical mucus interaction testing using a hyaluronate migration test. *Human Reproduction*, **5**: 835–41.

Mortimer, D., Aitken, R.J., Mortimer, S.T. & Pacey, A.A. (1995) Workshop report: clinical CASA – the quest for consensus. *Reproduction, Fertility and Development*, **7**: 951–9.

Neuwinger J., Behre, H. & Nieschlag, E. (1990) External quality control in the andrology laboratory: an experimental multicenter trial. *Fertility and Sterility*, **54**: 308–14.

Oehninger, S., Burkman, L.J., Coddington, C.C., Acosta, A.A., Scott, R., Franken, D.R. & Hodgen, G.D. (1989) Hemizona assay: assessment of sperm dysfunction and prediction of *in-vitro* fertilization outcome. *Fertility and Sterility*, **51**: 665–70.

Oei, S.G., Helmerhorst, F.M. & Keirse, M.J.N. (1995) When is the post-coital test normal? A critical appraisal. *Human Reproduction*, **10**: 1711–14.

*Ombelet, W., Menkveld, R., Kruger, T.F. & Steeno, O. (1995). Sperm morphology assessment: historical review in relation to fertility. *Human Reproduction*, **1**: 543–57.

Purvis, K. & Christiansen, E. (1993) Infection in the male reproductive tract. Impact, diagnosis and treatment in relation to male infertility. *International Journal of Andrology*, **16**: 1–13.

Rao, B., Soufir, J.C., Martin, M. & David, G. (1989) Lipid peroxidation in human spermatozoa as related to midpiece abnormalities and motility. *Gamete Research*, **24**: 127–34.

Rhemrev, J., Jeyendran, R.S., Vermeiden, J.P.W. & Zaneveld, L.J.D. (1989) Human sperm selection by glass wool filtration and two-layer discontinuous Percoll gradient centrifugation. *Fertility and Sterility*, **51**: 685–90.

Sbracia, M., Sayme, N., Grasso, J., Vigue, L. & Huszar, G. (1996) Sperm function and choice of preparation media: comparison of Percoll and Accudenz discontinuous density gradients. *Journal of Andrology*, **17**: 61–7.

Scarselli, G., Livi, C., Chelo, E., Dubini, V. & Pellagrini S. (1987) Approach to immunological male infertility: a comparison between MAR test and direct immunobead test. *Acta Europea Fertilitatis*, **18**: 55–9.

Smith, R., Vantman, D., Ponce, J., Escobar, J. & Lissi, E. (1996) Total antioxidant capacity of human seminal plasma. *Human Reproduction*, **11**: 1655–60.

Tomlinson, M.J., Barratt, C.L., Bolton, A.E., Lenton, E.A., Roberts, H.B. & Cooke, I.D. (1992) Round cells and sperm fertilizing capacity: the presence of immature germ cells but not seminal leukocytes are associated with reduced success of in vitro fertilization. *Fertility and Sterility*, **58**: 1257–9.

Tomlinson, M.J., Barratt, C.L.R. & Cooke, I.D. (1993) Prospective study of leukocytes and leukocyte subpopulations in semen suggests they are not a cause of male infertility. *Fertility and Sterility*, **60**: 1069–75.

von der Kammer, H., Scheit, K.H., Weidner, W. & Cooper, T.G. (1991) The evaluation of markers of prostatic function. *Urological Research*, **19**: 343–7.

Wolff, H., Politch, J.A., Martinez, A., Haimovici. F., Hill, J.A. & Anderson, D.J. (1990) Leukocytospermia is associated with poor semen quality. *Fertility and Sterility*, **53**: 528–36.

World Health Organization. (1983) *Laboratory Biosafety Manual*. pp. 1–123. Geneva: World Health Organization.

World Health Organization (1986) Consultation on the zona-free hamster oocyte penetration test and the diagnosis of male fertility. (ed. R.J. Aitken) *International Journal of Andrology (Supplement 6)*.

World Health Organization (1993) *Manual for the Standardized Investigation and Diagnosis of the Infertile Couple*. Cambridge: Cambridge University Press.

World Health Organization Task Force on Methods for the Regulation of Male Fertility (1990) Contraceptive efficacy of testosterone-induced azoospermia in normal men. *Lancet*, **336**: 995–9.

World Health Organization Task Force on Methods for the Regulation of Male Fertility (1996) Contraceptive efficacy of testosterone-induced azoospermia and oligozoospermia in normal men. *Fertility and Sterility*, **65**: 821–9.

Yanagimachi, R., Lopata, A., Odom, C.B., Bronson, R.A., Mahi, C.A. & Nicolson, A.L. (1979) Retention of biologic characteristics of zona pellucida in highly concentrated salt solution: the use of salt stored eggs for assessing the fertilizing capacity of spermatozoa. *Fertility and Sterility*, **31**: 562–74.

Yeung, C.H., Cooper, T.G. & Nieschlag, E. (1997) A technique for standardisation and quality control of subjective sperm motility assessments in semen analysis. *Fertility and Sterility*, **67**: 1156–8.

de Ziegler, D., Cedars, M.I., Hamilton, F., Moreno, T. & Meldrum, D.R. (1987) Factors influencing maintenance of sperm motility during in vitro processing. *Fertility and Sterility*, **48**: 816–20.

Zinaman, M.J., Uhler, M.L., Vertuno, E., Fisher, S.G. & Clegg, E.D. (1996) Evaluation of computer-assisted semen analysis (CASA) with IDENT stain to determine sperm concentration. *Journal of Andrology*, **17**: 288–92.

# Index